# Foundations in Nursing and Health Care

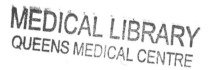

# Beginning Reflective Practice

**Melanie Jasper**

Series Editor: Lynne Wigens

## Nelson Thornes

Published in 2003 by:
Nelson Thornes Ltd
Delta Place
27 Bath Road
CHELTENHAM
GL53 7TH
United Kingdom

08 / 10 9 8

A catalogue record for this book is available from the British Library

ISBN 978 0 7487 7117 2

Illustrations by Clinton Banbury
Page make-up by Michael Fay

Printed in Croatia by Zrinski

# Contents

*1005863134*

# Acknowledgements

The author would like to acknowledge the following for their support and encouragement:

The students and colleagues that have provided the inspiration and many of the practical applications for this book.

My dear friend and colleague Gary Rolfe, without whom I would never have written a word all those years ago, and who continues to offer opportunities that I cannot refuse. My mentor Neil Lindfield, who has always provided unfailing, thoughtful and encouraging support, reins in my wilder tendencies and tolerates my flights of fancy. Chris and Anna, who accept their mother as she is; and Andrew, who has made a significant contribution to this book, did he but know it!

The author and publishers would also like to thank the following for permission to reproduce material in this book:

Routledge (Sharples 1999) p. 57 and Blackwell Scientific (Johns 2000) p. 97.

Every effort has been made to contact other copyright holders and the publishers apologise to anyone whose rights have been inadvertently overlooked and will be happy to rectify any errors or omissions.

# Introduction

In this book we introduce you to the concept of reflective practice – what it is and why it is important both as a strategy for your own learning and for developing your professional practice. The purpose of this introduction is to set the scene of reflective practice for you. You can then approach the rest of the book with an understanding of what you are trying to achieve in developing strategies for your own learning from practice experiences. We also use this section to introduce the rest of the book to you.

None of us comes to learning as a blank slate; we all have a wealth of knowledge and experiences that form a springboard for developing new and exciting roles and skills. As a fledgling professional, you will be faced with what might, at the moment, seem like a daunting array and amount of learning. This comes firstly from both the hard slog of learning facts and accepted knowledge, and secondly from acquiring and practising the physical skills of your profession with confidence so that they become second nature. As you start to tick these off your list, though, you will find that other elements of professional practice start to creep into your consciousness. You will meet professional codes of conduct, and ethics. These underpin the ways in which we form relationships with our clients and enable us to do things to them that under other circumstances would be seen as beyond normal interaction with strangers – things such as touching, or asking personal questions, or expecting people to reveal parts of their bodies to us that would normally remain covered. Many of these areas will be considered by looking at how you communicate with others and explaining how to form professional relationships that are 'common knowledge' because of the unspoken boundaries accepted by both the professional and the client.

We can often only learn these things by observing others, being placed in the situation ourselves and building up experiences that we can draw on.

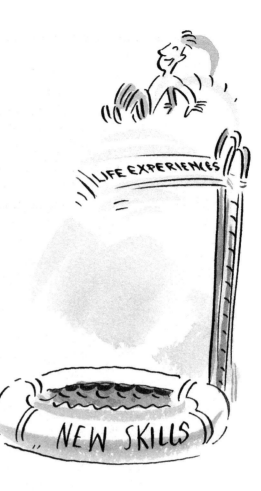

*All our experiences act as a springboard for developing new skills*

And this is where reflective practice comes in. The ideas and strategies that you meet in this book are designed to help you become aware of this professional development in the third area of knowledge and skills. You will need these skills when you finally graduate from your course and are entitled to be called a professional. Reflective skills, particularly structured reflective strategies, enable us to make the most of everything that we do. This includes not only remembering things that have already happened but also anticipating and planning for the future.

In Chapter 1, 'What is reflective practice?', we set the scene of reflective practice, exploring what it is and why we need it as a strategy for learning from our professional experience. We introduce you to the basic theories underpinning reflective practice and explore the key concepts within it in detail. This chapter provides you with the foundation for understanding what reflective practice is and why it is important.

In Chapter 2, 'Knowing ourselves', we start you off using reflective techniques. The first section in this chapter will help you identify your own strengths and weaknesses and start you thinking about how you can make the most of these as you proceed through your course. In the second section we ask you to think about the professional values that will underpin your practice, and where these come from. The next section looks at your learning style, with the last section identifying your approaches to writing. These last two sections will help you think about the ways in which you learn most effectively, and how you can plan to use these through your course and in your continuing development as a practitioner.

Chapter 3, 'Frameworks for reflection', presents three frameworks for reflective practice that can be used to structure your reflective activities. These are fully illustrated to help you see concrete examples of the ways in which they have helped other students to learn. These are fundamental in reflective practice as they provide a starting point for understanding what reflective cycles and processes involve. They provide a useful initial structure for reflective activities that you may then decide to build upon in the future.

In Chapter 4, 'Entering the clinical environment', we explore your role within the clinical environment and how you can use reflective practice to learn in it. Clinical environments offer you unique experiences that, unlike classroom learning, need to be explored and reinforced if we are to learn from them. It is easy to go through a day in practice without acknowledging the learning experiences that occur or ensuring that you identify your achievements. This chapter looks at maximising your learning opportunities and making the most of what is available in different environments.

Chapter 5, 'Ways of reflecting on your own', and Chapter 6, 'Ways of reflecting with others', consider the different ways in which you can reflect by yourself or with other people. We look in depth at the advantages and challenges to both approaches, and raise issues to help you to explore the ways in which you can create opportunities and strategies for reflection. Chapter 5 focuses on strategies that you can use by yourself and includes sections on working with your learning style and thinking through your experiences. Most of the reflection you do will be by yourself and will not occur in a formal way at all. We try to get you thinking about how you can acknowledge this reflective work, whether it occurs while you are in practice or after the event. The majority of this chapter is devoted to exploring strategies for reflective writing in some depth. The purpose of this is to help you to think about your own attitudes about writing and to plan to use writing as a way of learning for yourself.

Chapter 6 focuses on the strategies that you can use when reflecting with others, especially those whose role it is to help you in your learning, such as your supervisors and lecturers. Reflecting with others has a different character from reflecting by yourself because you are essentially making your own unique experiences public. Reflecting with others is very powerful as a strategy for learning because you are able to draw on the perspectives that others bring to a situation. But this brings with it roles and responsibilities for all concerned to ensure that reflection is carried out in safety. This chapter identifies the issues that need to be considered before starting a reflective relationship with another person, so that maximum benefit can be gained by all those involved.

## Using this book to develop skills for reflective practice

Throughout the book we will be providing you with tips and pointers so that the decisions you make about your own reflective practice can be informed ones that you make consciously. We present the issues that you need to consider about each of the topics covered, in the hope that this will enable you to use reflective techniques effectively as a strategy for your own learning.

This book aims to be both an introduction to reflective practice and a practical guide to help you to develop strategies and skills to begin your career as a reflective practitioner. Reflective practice is a technique for learning from experience that is applicable to all students in health-care professions. We have used a range of examples throughout the book to illustrate the ideas being presented to you. Some of these arise from specific disciplines, such as nursing or physiotherapy, while others are the sorts of thing that could happen to anyone. The purpose of using examples from practice is to show you how a raw experience can be used as data for analysis and reflection to help you to learn and take action. The focus of the example itself is therefore not really relevant. So, if you are a student operating department practitioner, for instance, use the examples for the general point they are trying to convey rather than for the discipline they are drawn from.

Reflective practice is a deliberate activity – you have to take a decision to focus *deliberately* on something specific in order to learn from it. Throughout this book you will find a range of activities designed to help you develop the skills and strategies for reflective practice, by actually doing it. To get the most out of this book, it is worth taking the time to pick up pen and paper, or find other people to reflect with, while you work through the activities. Although reading the book will help you explore and understand what reflective practice is, the bottom line is that you can only learn from doing it yourself – there will be no miraculous transmission of skills, strategies and ideas from this book to your head! So, even if you are tempted to skip over the activities, do read them through and think about what they are asking you to do. At least come up with skeleton answers, even if you do not want to commit them to paper in the first instance.

In this book we take the approach that learning is not a passive exercise. We assume that the most effective and enjoyable way to learn from written material is to interact with what you are reading. So, we offer you several different ways of doing this, as we ask you to play with the ideas and consider what you are reading in the light of your own experiences.

First, in each of the chapters you will meet **case studies** that have been taken from students' real life experiences. These will illustrate the issues that the chapter is dealing with, and show how reflective practice can occur in a range of diverse examples. The intention of the case studies is to demonstrate how the theories designed to be appropriate to everyone can be applied to specific individual cases to provide understanding and facilitate learning. By engaging with these examples you will see how the ideas presented translate into other people's experiences and help them to make a bit more sense of what has happened to them.

Second, there are sections called '**reflective activity**' at key stages through each chapter. These give you time to reflect on the ideas that you are meeting and relate them in some way to your own experiences. As a result, you will be engaging in reflective activities and building up the skills for reflective practice as you go. As with most skills, the more we do them the better we get, and we hope that by introducing them to you gradually, and getting you to think about what has happened to you, or others around you, you will start to include them in the way that you learn almost automatically. We will also ask you to think about how useful the activities are to you, how you felt about doing them, and how effective they were in helping you understand your experiences. So, these exercises operate at two levels. Firstly, they will be asking you to do something that will help you to understand the ideas that are being presented and how they relate to you. Secondly, you will be analysing and evaluating the strategies at a deeper level, so that you recognise the usefulness of the strategy as a tool in itself. This will enable you to select those approaches that fit best with the way that you like to work and learn.

Third, throughout the book we identify **key words**. You will meet new terms, ideas and words as you read. Many of these will be defined in the margin for you, to help you to 'translate' the word for your own use so that you become comfortable with using the words and the concepts that they incorporate.

Fourth, we go '**over to you**' and ask you to think about how what you have just read relates to you and your experiences. You may be asked to think about what you will actually do with what you have just learned or discovered.

Fifth, we offer you some **key points** at the end of sections to remind you of the main points made or provide a summary of the ideas that have been presented.

Finally, we offer you an opportunity to test your understanding of the key issues raised by asking you **rapid recap** questions at the end of each chapter. The answers to these will be found at the end of the book.

We hope that you will enjoy learning to be a reflective practitioner with the help of the ideas and techniques presented through this book. It aims to be a practical guide and introduction to reflective practice for those starting out on the road of becoming health-care practitioners. We wish you success in your learning and in your future career in working with other people to improve their lives and their experience of the health-care system.

# 1

# What is reflective practice?

## Learning outcomes

By the end of this chapter you should be able to:

- Begin to understand the concept of reflective practice
- Distinguish between reflective processes and reflective practice
- Appreciate how reflection can be seen as a strategy for learning
- Understand how learning can occur from experience
- Recognise opportunities for learning within a practice/clinical environment
- Understand how reflective practice can help to bridge theory and practice

Reflective practice has been identified as one of the key ways in which we can learn from our experiences. In education for health-care professions it is recognised as an essential tool for helping students to make the links between theory and practice. It enables you to develop your knowledge and skills towards becoming professional practitioners. Essentially, reflective practice means taking our experiences as a starting point for learning. By thinking about them in a purposeful way – using the reflective processes – we can come to understand them differently and take action as a result. The learning that we achieve using reflective strategies is different from the theory that provides the knowledge underpinning our practice. It is also different from acquiring skills by watching others and mimicking what they do, because it involves consciously thinking about things and actively making decisions. Hence, reflective practice bridges the gap between pure theory and directed practice by providing a strategy that helps to develop understanding and learning.

Much of the work during your course will concentrate on providing you with the knowledge for evidence-based practice and enabling you to develop the practical skills necessary to reach the standards for registration as a practitioner. However, there is a third element that you need to work on. It integrates the other two and helps you to become a responsible professional practitioner, aware of your own knowledge and skills, and your limitations, so that you are both competent and safe. This third area is complex, because it involves developing the critical analytical skills and judgement that allow you to make decisions, and can only arise from encountering different situations in the real world of practice. One of the most important ways you will do this is through reflective practice. The skills learned during the foundations of your professional training will stay with you, becoming part of who you are as a practitioner. This is probably the most significant way that you will actually practise once you have qualified.

## What is reflective practice?

Reflective practice as a **concept** for learning was introduced into many professions in the 1980s. It is seen as one of the ways that professionals learn from experience in order to understand and develop their practice. The idea behind this is a relatively simple one. Basically, reflective practice means that we learn by thinking about things that have happened to us and seeing them in a different way, which enables us to take some kind of action.

Reflective practice can be summarised as having three components:

- Things (experiences) that happen to a person
- The reflective processes that enable the person to learn from those experiences
- The action that results from the new perspectives that are taken.

These can be summarised as experience–reflection–action (ERA) and seen as a cycle (Figure 1.1).

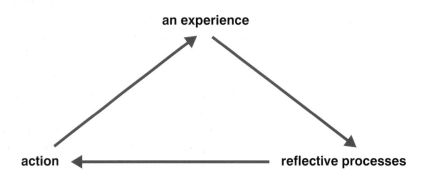

**Figure 1.1** *The ERA cycle of reflective practice*

However, this could remain as a series of separate events unless thought about as a process through which we actively learn. The idea of reflection as a learning process arises from educational theorists such as Dewey (1938), who suggested that 'we learn by doing and realising what came of what we did', and has been developed by many others since then. One key figure is Kolb (1984), who developed what he called a cycle of **experiential learning**, which has formed the basis of many strategies (sometimes called *models*) for reflective practice in the past two decades.

Kolb's work is often referred to as presenting the foundations for learning from experience, as he describes a cycle of stages that we go through, shown in Figure 1.2.

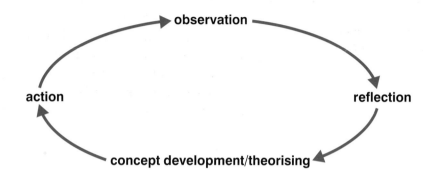

**Figure 1.2** *Kolb's experiential learning cycle (1984)*

Basically, he draws attention to the fact that, when we want to learn from something that has already happened to us, we need to recall our observations of the event and then reflect on those observations in some way. We do this through reflective processes that ask us to describe the experience and analyse it so that, at the end, we form some ideas or theories about it. As a result of these reflections we will come to a deeper understanding of what has happened and will therefore develop our own theories or concepts about it. Once we have these ideas in our heads, Kolb suggests that we frame some action as a result and that this possible course of action is seen as our 'learning'. This will then inform any action that we take as a result of the experience.

The cyclical nature of reflective practice is the key to moving forward as practitioners, in that we rarely stop at just the one cycle. If we complete the first cycle, i.e. we *consciously* take action as a result of the reflective processes we have undertaken, then the next time we have that experience, or one similar to it, we will encounter it in a different way. Thus, the experience itself has been transformed, making it into a different experience. So, if we go through the cycle again, we are building our knowledge and understanding of it each time. This can be seen as a continual spiral incorporating several reflective cycles, as shown in Figure 1.3.

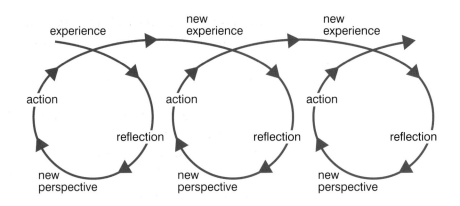

**Figure 1.3** *A reflective spiral*

Reflective learning, then, is not simply a matter of thinking about something that has already happened as a retrospective activity. It can also be seen as a predictive activity: as a strategy for planning our learning for the future on the basis of what we already know and on what we can anticipate. Guiding the whole reflective process is the desire to come to a deeper understanding about something that has happened to us. In order to do this we need to be open to different ways of looking at our experiences in order to develop as practitioners.

**Key points** Top tips

- Reflective practice is a strategy that we can use to learn from our practice
- It consists of the ERA cycle (experience, reflection, action)

## Why do we reflect?

We engage in reflective activity for a number of reasons. Perhaps the most basic is the need for us to develop strategies for survival throughout our lives. An inability to build life skills as a result of learning from our experiences puts us at risk. For instance, think of the care and attention that small children need to keep them safe when outside, or the problems that people who suffer from dementia have as a result of 'forgetting' the fundamental lessons of safety in daily life.

Although most of us have developed reflective strategies to ensure that we do learn as a result of what happens to us, on the whole we would not regard this as a fundamental way in which we have built up our knowledge and skills. It is only when we are asked to consider the ways in which we learn best, and identify how we know what it is that we know, that we start to consciously think about how we learn throughout life. The ways in which you have come to be the person you are and the ways in which you learn will be explored in Chapter 2. However, it is worth identifying briefly here the purposes for which we use reflective strategies for learning from our experiences in professional practice. We might use them in the following ways:

- To identify learning needs
- To identify new opportunities for learning
- To identify the ways in which we learn best
- To identify new courses of action
- To explore alternative ways of solving problems
- For personal development
- For professional development
- To escape routine practice
- To be aware of the consequences of our actions
- To demonstrate our competence to others
- To demonstrate our achievements to ourselves and others
- To build theory from observations
- To help us make decisions or resolve uncertainty
- To empower or emancipate ourselves as individuals.

## Types of reflection

For the purposes of this book, we are going to divide reflection into two types – reflection-in-action and reflection-on-action. These were identified by Donald Schön (1983) as the principal ways that professionals use to conceptualise and articulate their knowledge.

### Reflection-in-action

Reflection-in-action is the way that people think and theorise about practice while they are doing it. This is often seen as an automatic activity that occurs subconsciously in practice at an everyday level. It is perceived by some people to be intuitive and an 'unconscious' process, and therefore not really reflective activity that we use deliberately. It is often seen as the way that advanced practitioners

⚷ *Keywords*

**Cognitive**
Involving thoughtful,
conscious understanding

practise, as a result of the combination of their knowledge, skills and practice. This is not to say that we don't all use reflection-in-action to some degree when practising, as we sift through alternatives and choose to do what we do without really being aware that we are doing it. Examples of this are when we use our interpersonal skills in a facilitative way, such as persuading an immobile patient to walk to the washroom, or deciding which pressure-relieving device to use for a particular patient.

## Reflection-on-action

Reflection-on-action involves us in consciously exploring experience and thinking about practice after it has occurred to discover the knowledge used in the situation. It occurs through analysis, interpretation and the recombination of information about the experience so that new perspectives are found about what has happened. This usually happens retrospectively and away from the scene of practice. And it assumes that practice is underpinned by knowledge and is thus a **cognitive** process. Reflection-on-action can therefore be seen as an *active* process of transforming experience into knowledge and involves much more than simply thinking about and describing practice. Examples of this may be a student sitting down with a staff nurse to talk through cardiac arrest procedure after she has witnessed it, or a case discussion between a student and clinical supervisor that involves reviewing the student's work with the patient and planning resultant action.

We will be focussing on reflection-on-action throughout this book, as we are considering the conscious development of strategies for reflective practice as learning from and for practice. However, Rolfe and colleagues (2001) explore the concept of reflection-in-action further in their book *Critical Reflection for Nursing and the Helping Professions* in relation to the ways that practitioners, particularly at an advanced level, may be using reflective strategies as part of their everyday practice.

## Levels of reflection

Goodman (1984) suggests that there are three levels of reflection that a reflective practitioner may achieve. These are shown in Table 1.1.

| Table 1.1  **Goodman's levels of reflection (1984)** |
| --- |
| **1st level**<br>**Reflection to reach given objectives** – criteria for reflection are limited to technocratic issues of efficiency, effectiveness and accountability |
| **2nd level**<br>**Reflection on the relationship between principles and practice** – there is an assessment of the implications and consequences of actions and beliefs as well as the underlying rationale for practice |
| **3rd level**<br>**Reflection which besides the above incorporates ethical and political concerns** – issues of justice and emancipation enter the deliberations over the value of professional goals and practice and the practitioner makes links between the setting of everyday practice and broader social structure and forces. |

As a student you will be expected to work your way up through these gradually, beginning with the first level, which is mainly descriptive. As you move through your course, becoming more familiar with the strategies used in reflective practice and more comfortable with your skills and knowledge, you will also be expected to start using the second and third levels. These help you to explore the complex incidents and situations that you encounter in practice by considering drawing on theoretical perspectives and evidence – the personal and professional aspects and the ethical and political issues that are a feature of the society in which we live.

Goodman's levels are explored further, and illustrated, in Chapter 3.

**Key points** Top tips

- Reflection can be used for a number of different purposes
- There are two types of reflection – reflection-in-action and reflection-on-action
- Goodman identified three levels of reflection

## The ERA components

It is worth taking some more time here to establish what we mean by the three ERA components. Remember, ERA stands for 'experience–reflection–action'. These form the foundation on which you will build your knowledge and skills for reflective practice and it is therefore important that you understand their principles. All strategies for reflection use these three components in different ways and use different words to describe them – but the underlying principles remain the same.

## The nature of experience

### What is experience?

There are several different ways that we can look at the idea of experience. First, we might say 'I had an exciting experience the other day'. Used in this way, the word 'experience' means something that has happened to us that we are aware of through our senses and can describe. For instance, this might have been a visit to a particular place or a meeting with someone. We might refer to this as 'an' experience and are using the word as a noun to mean something in itself. This suggests that we ourselves have taken part in the experience and therefore have first hand knowledge of it.

Second, we may say 'She has a lot of experience in counselling distressed teenagers', in which case we are referring to an accumulation of knowledge and skill built up over time in a particular area. This will also mean the totality of the experiences a person has had.

Finally, we might say 'I experienced something strange yesterday', in which case we are using the word as a verb, something that we 'do' or have done. In this sense, 'to experience something' means that we have done it or gone through it.

The CancerWeb Dictionary (2000) describes experience as:

> *the feeling of emotions and sensations, as opposed to thinking; involvement in what is happening rather than abstract reflection on an event or interpersonal encounter.*

An important distinction for reflective practice is made in this definition, in that experience is seen as something very practical. It is the 'doing' or 'feeling' of something rather than any thoughts about it.

When we use the term 'experience' in this book, it is this definition that we will be referring to.

So we may talk about:

- *An* experience as something that has happened to you
- The *accumulation of knowledge and skills* over time, or
- The *processes* that you go though when you do something.

In addition to these components of experience, some dictionaries also suggest that experience in itself leads to learning. For instance, Webster's Dictionary (2000) sees experience as:

> an act of knowledge, one or more by which single facts or general truths are ascertained; experimental or inductive knowledge; hence implying skill, facility or practical wisdom gained by personal knowledge, feeling or action.

And Wordnet 1.6 (1997) says that experience is:

> the accumulation of knowledge or skill that results from direct participation in events or activities.

So the first-hand experiences that we have as the basis for learning within practice settings are fundamental to the concept of reflective practice.

When we talk about experience, or experiences, in this book, we mean anything that might have happened to you in the past. This does not necessarily have to be related to, or to have arisen from, your professional field. In fact, very often we learn a great deal about ourselves by exploring how we act in one setting, recognising the ways we do this and deliberately transferring that strategy to unfamiliar situations. We will be using many of your past experiences in this way later in the book, to help you recognise the ways in which you deal with the world and the many different things that are thrown at you in life. From these you will come to understand how you react in different circumstances and what ways you already have of coping with the world. You will also be presented with others to help you to develop further in your professional roles.

However, we can go through the whole of our lives having experiences and not necessarily learn from them or, at least, not being aware that we have learned from them. Fundamental to the concept of reflective practice is that we *consciously* or *knowingly* consider our experiences in order to draw out our learning. Hence, learning from experience becomes a deliberate act, rather than it happening by accident.

---

### Reflective activity

Make two lists of the things that you have done over the past week. On one side of the page write down 10 things that you would consider to be routine, or regular experiences. In this list might be things like 'catching the bus to college'; 'collecting the children from school'; 'doing the weekly shopping'. Your second list will be 10 things that have been different from your usual experiences, and probably stick out more in your mind because of this – for instance, you may have booked a holiday, been to a party, received a piece of work back from a tutor or learned a new skill at work.

Select one of the experiences in your first list, and think about how you did it. Ask yourself the following questions:

● What did I do?

● Why did I do it the way I did?

● What other ways could I have done it?

● How did I know to do it the way I did?

● What had I learned from doing it previously that means that I did it the way I did?

Now repeat this using an experience from your second list, answering these extra questions as well:

● What experience, or previous learning, have I drawn on to inform this experience?

● What new learning has occurred?

● What have I learned that I will be able to use in the future?

---

How often do we take time to sit down and consider our everyday experiences and think about just how it is that we come to do as we do? In fact, how often do we really know what it is that we do? We tend to go through most of our days in a routine way that enables us to pack into our time all the things that we need to, often without thinking about them. In fact, if we did think about them, there's a chance that we'd never get anything done at all, because we'd be slowed up by consciously having to think about everything we do. It is even possible that we would not be as efficient at what we do, simply because we are thinking about it! For instance, people who drive a car regularly do not think about the mechanics of driving; they do it automatically so that they can concentrate on the driving conditions and respond to the circumstances they are in. If they were thinking about every gear change or clutch depression, it is likely that they would drive dangerously because their full attention would not be on the road. It is also highly likely that the quality of their driving would deteriorate because cognitive processes were interfering with what had become instinctive practice. An illustration of this is the insecurity that can arise when we have to drive in a country that uses the other side of the road or where the road signs and rules of driving are different, and we have to think more carefully about what we are doing.

In looking back at your answers to the exercise, can you identify elements of this happening to you in the first example that you used? How much of your efficiency is due to the fact that the way you do something has become ingrained, so much so that you are unaware of how you are doing it? Yet, at one time, you were not this efficient – you have built the ability up through repetition and things have become second nature. It does not even occur to you to do things differently unless you consciously make a decision to think of alternatives. This often happens as a result of watching someone else do the same thing, but in a different way from ourselves. For instance, you might watch the way another person does a task and think 'What are they doing it like that for? It's much easier the way I do it!', or perhaps the opposite, that they seem to achieve a better or quicker result than you. As a result, you might decide to change the way that you do it yourself.

In the second example that you used, you may have found that you were more conscious of what you were doing at the time you were doing it, and therefore found it easier to answer the questions. It is in unfamiliar situations, or those that occur less frequently, that we tend to think consciously about what we are doing. Perhaps we then refer to the rules that we have learned, or drag explanations out from our subconscious in order to make decisions and take action – or to be able to justify that action. For instance, if you are booking a holiday, you will be actively drawing on your previous experiences in order to make decisions about the future – things such as whether to use a travel agent or book through the Internet, the type of place you want to go and the type of accommodation that will suit your needs, and the amount of money that you have to spend. Other things that will occur to you may involve checking your passport, booking your dog into kennels and ordering a taxi to take you to the airport. Other people focus on preparing the house so that it is secure, and hiding valuables.

None of these considerations happen either automatically or by accident. They come into your mind as a result of thoughtful processes that draw on your previous experiences of booking a holiday, or on experiences with similar features that enable you to apply what you have learned from one situation to another. It is this deliberate activity of using reflective processes to explore our experiences that enables us to identify, acknowledge and value our experiential learning. We need to know more about these reflective processes in order to use them effectively to learn from our experiences.

---

**Key points** | Top tips

- Everything that happens to us can be seen as an experience that can be reflected on and learned from
- We can transfer our learning from one experience into others
- We need to consciously use our experiences as the starting point of our learning

---

## What are reflective processes?

Reflective processes help us to see the world in alternative ways by enabling us to focus on different aspects of our experiences. By reflective processes we mean the stages of thoughtful activity that we go through when we consciously decide to explore an experience. There are many ways in which we can reflect, and a variety of strategies for doing this are discussed in Chapter 3. In this section however, we want to outline the basic ideas behind using a structure for reflecting that run throughout all the strategies you will meet later, whether you are reflecting by yourself or with other people.

The fundamental stages of the reflective processes are:

- Stage 1: Selecting a critical incident to reflect on
- Stage 2: Observing and describing the experience
- Stage 3: Analysing the experience
- Stage 4: Interpreting the experience
- Stage 5: Exploring alternatives
- Stage 6: Framing action.

### Stage 1: Selecting a critical incident to reflect on

**The critical incident**

As we have seen in the previous section, any experience that we have can be used as a focus for reflection. However, what we choose to reflect on needs to have some significance for us, in terms of what we are trying to achieve or the purpose that it is going to serve. When reflecting for learning as part of a course, we need to identify events that will contribute to our learning as a developing practitioner; therefore these events need to be significant in some way.

**Keywords**

**Critical incident**
Event that stands out in
your mind and contributes
directly to development
as a practitioner

Throughout this book, we will refer to these events as **critical incidents**. This term was first coined in 1954 by John Flanagan, a psychologist working with the US Air Force. He defined it in the following way:

> *By an incident is meant any observable human activity that is sufficiently complete in itself to permit inferences and predictions to be made about the person performing the act. To be critical, an incident must occur in a situation where the purpose or intent of the act seems fairly clear to the observer and where its consequences are sufficiently definite to leave little doubt concerning its effects.*
>
> Flanagan 1954, p. 327

To simplify this: we can see that critical incidents are episodes of experience that have particular meaning to the observer, practitioner or any other person taking part in them. They may be positive or negative experiences and must be suitable for being described in a concise way. Critical incidents are usually seen as something that has already happened to us but in this book we want to broaden that definition in terms of anticipating the future. While we are not expecting you to have a crystal ball, as a student there is a certain degree of predictability about the experiences you will have during your course. By reflecting on what is coming up, in terms of clinical placements or college work, you can anticipate your learning needs and plan to use your time more effectively. Similarly, you will have been given learning outcomes for your course, and all disciplines will have practical skills or competencies that need to be achieved before you can be licensed to practise your profession. So, in terms of the subject matter for reflective practice and learning, thinking about what you need to achieve is as significant as thinking about any of the experiences you have already had.

When a critical incident is significant, it sticks in our minds for a number of reasons. These may be because it made us feel good or valued, or that we felt we were doing a good job or had achieved success at something. It may also be because it made us feel angry or dejected or devalued in some way. We might also feel that negative consequences were our fault, or a result of actions we took that were somehow wrong, or that we made a mistake that has resulted in someone suffering. Other examples might be a comment you made to someone that was taken in a different way from the one in which it was meant, and a row exploded, or that you hear that someone is saying things about you that you think are unfair or untrue. Unfortunately, the term 'critical incident' has often been misunderstood within the context of reflective practice. Part of the reason for this lies in the fact that we are working in health-care professions where the word 'critical' is often used to mean 'serious'. If we go back to Flanagan's definition, though, we can see that this was not the original intention. Flanagan meant 'critical' to mean something that stands out in some way, and this is the way in which we will be using the term in this book. Another confusion that has crept into the idea of reflective strategies has been the idea that all stimuli for reflection come from critical incidents that have caused us uncomfortable feelings or discomfort in some way. This notion arose in a paper by Atkins and Murphy (1993), who suggested that we have a need to reflect from:

> *an awareness of uncomfortable feelings or thoughts. This arises from a realisation that, in a situation, the knowledge one was applying was not sufficient in itself to explain what was happening in that unique situation.*
>
> Atkins and Murphy 1993, p. 1189

While undoubtedly much reflection is stimulated by unpleasant or uncomfortable feelings, this one notion of reflection has spread to such an extent within nursing as to provide a negative connotation for the whole process. Many practitioners have been introduced to the reflective process through the idea that reflective practice arises solely from things that have caused discomfort. Atkins and Murphy's intention was not to direct the course of reflective practice through a focus on things that caused us concern! The origins of the paper were in a literature review identifying the state of reflective practice at the time of writing. Since then, many authors and practitioners have developed the ideas of reflective practice and turned the underpinning features around to enable the term to encompass all our 'critical incidents', whether positive or negative. Of course, when you think about it logically, we tend to build on success. In the past many of us unconsciously repeated actions and ways of working that had previously been successful and avoided ones that had not. The overt use of reflective processes, and critical reflection at that, is to enable us to learn deliberatively from our experiences and to identify action that can be taken in the future.

Sources for reflection can therefore come from any experience we have had, and we can learn from things that have gone well just as effectively as from negative experiences. In fact, the reason that we tend to dwell on things that go wrong is that for most of the time everything in our lives goes well, and we take this for granted!

## Reflective activity

Think back over the previous week and list all the things that have happened to you that you felt didn't turn out as you wanted them to.

Now make a list of everything that went successfully.

How long is the second list in comparison to the first one?

We don't tend to give ourselves much credit for everyday things that go right – getting to college on time, for instance, or ensuring that there is enough bread and milk in the house for breakfast. But, if these things don't happen, we are likely to remember and take steps to prevent the situation from occurring again. One reason for this is a natural instinct to avoid situations that will cause us stress and make us feel uncomfortable. We learn to take things that go right in our stride and not to focus on them; as a result we do not give ourselves credit for our part in them. Hence, when something does go wrong, whether it is our fault or not, we tend to blame ourselves and feel guilty and uncomfortable. It is a natural drive to want to avoid these stressful feelings, so we reflect on what has happened in order to learn from the experience and change our behaviour.

In the early days of the use of reflective processes in health-care education, students were encouraged to focus on events that had caused them to feel uncomfortable in some way (Atkins and Murphy 1993). As a result, many practitioners perceived experiential learning negatively and associated it with reminders of where they felt inadequate or to blame in some way. However, this focus has changed as reflective processes have developed into mainstream techniques for learning in courses, and apply to all the outcomes that need to be achieved by students. Hence, reflective processes are now used not only to learn from things that have already happened but also to plan learning experiences to fulfil identified needs on the basis of the experiences we have already had. Some universities are now using reflective practice as the main strategy for learning in their health-care courses, incorporating within it the other learning and teaching strategies used previously.

We can see, therefore, that the selection of experiences has become important in ensuring that students are able to maximise the learning that they achieve. In addition to identifying an experience solely for reasons of what you can learn from it, there are other issues to take into account.

**The other people involved**

As a student health-care practitioner, it is unlikely that you will be working in isolation. Hence, in the majority of experiences other people will be involved, ranging from the patients you are caring for, their relatives and other carers to your fellow students and colleagues, supervisors, other practitioners and educational staff.

You may need to consider all the other people involved, both as part of the experience itself and in the reflective activity.

The type of event involving other people that you choose to reflect on will depend on whether your reflective activity is going to be shared with other people. Will others be involved in exploring the case with you or reading a reflective account of it? If you are choosing the event solely for your own purposes, and the results of your reflections will be kept private, you do not have to worry about any far-reaching consequences of what you are doing. However, if the event is to be shared with others you need to take into account several issues. These are covered in more detail in Chapter 6 and are simply summarised here as markers.

When focusing on events involving other people you need to think about:

- The effect that this might have on the other people involved
- Gaining consent from the others involved
- The status of any written records that you might make
- Confidentiality and protecting others.

When considering reflecting with others in a professional context, think about:

- The contextual implications of discussing things that have happened
- Choosing what to tell and considering the implications of this
- Working within professional codes of conduct and discussing the implications of this
- The consequences of disclosure
- Misconduct/malpractice/negligence
- Understanding the responsibilities of others within their professional role.

**Establishing the purpose of your reflective activity**

Finally, the reasons why you are reflecting will affect what it is that you choose to reflect on, and several of these were outlined on page 5. Establishing the purpose of your reflection will help you to select from the experiences available and match up the experience with the outcome.

| Key points | Top tips |

- Experiences for reflection can come from a multitude of sources, such as:
  - Any part of your life
  - Things that have gone well
  - Things that make you happy
  - Things that you feel uncomfortable about
  - Things that have made you sad
  - Things that have gone wrong
  - Observations that other people have made about you
  - Your relationships with others
- Selecting an experience to reflect on depends on:
  - The purpose of your reflection, i.e. why you are doing it
  - Who else may be part of the experience or incident,
    e.g. patients, carers, other professional staff
  - Who else may be part of the reflective process,
    i.e. talking or reading about your experiences
  - The possible consequences
- All experiences can be seen as *critical incidents* because they stick in our mind in some way and contribute to our professional development
- When choosing an incident to reflect on it is important to consider the roles that other people played in it
- It is important to identify the purpose of reflecting on the incident chosen

## Stage 2: Observing and describing the experience

The purpose of this stage of the reflective process is to produce as full a description of your experience as possible. It is helpful, especially when you are beginning reflective practice, to use a framework of key questions to structure the description of your experiences. These help you to focus on the essential structure of what happened and ensure that you consider all aspects of it. Some of these frameworks are explored and illustrated in Chapter 3.

A useful *aide memoire* for guiding this and the next two stages of the ERA cycle is what has come to be known as the **six wise men**.

These are the words that start the questions that you will be asking, and are worth committing to memory to help you start reflective practice. They are:

- Who
- What
- Where
- When
- Why
- How

These are used for training journalists to take down the key elements of a story that they are reporting on, so that they don't miss anything out. The first four will be used in the descriptive phase, whereas you will use the 'why' and 'how' questions in the analytical and interpretive phases as you come to understand more deeply what has happened. They do not necessarily need to be used in this order, however. As you become more familiar with strategies for reflective practice you will find that you re-order the ways in which you use the cue questions to suit the experience you are reflecting on and the purpose you want it to achieve.

This will provide the basic record of the event and the data that you use as raw material for the later stages. You can either do this verbally or create a written record.

### To write or not to write?

You have the choice of writing, or not writing, the description of your experiences. Written reflection has a different character to contemplative or verbal reflection, and detailed consideration is given to this in Chapter 5. In this you will explore the features of written reflection by looking at:

- The reason why we write
- How we can use writing to help order our thoughts
- The purpose of creating a permanent record
- How we can be creative through writing
- Using writing to develop our analytical skills
- Using writing to develop our critical thinking
- Using writing to develop new understandings and knowledge
- Using writing to show that we understand
- Writing in the first person (i.e. writing 'I went', 'I felt')

Do remember that your memory of an event will change over time, as our minds select what they consider to be the most significant parts of the experience to suit their purpose at any given time. For instance, close to a traumatic event, you will concentrate on your emotional reactions, as these enable you to deal with the situation and to take action to prevent yourself from being harmed. Therefore, you are likely to focus on the cause of your distress and attempt to justify your reactions and feelings. Later, however, when you are feeling safer, your mind will allow you to think more widely, and perhaps more rationally, about the situation, and therefore your reflections will be different. Written records bring benefits here, in that they allow you to record and then revisit your records as many times as you want after the events. This is something that reflecting verbally may not offer you: it may be restricted to a particular occasion and person that might not be available at a later date. Verbal reflection also takes place at a particular time, whether close to the event or at some other stage. Again, this brings its own benefits and drawbacks, and these are considered in Chapter 5.

**Key points**  Top tips

- The purpose of the description is to get as full a picture of what happened as possible
- The 'six wise men' can be used as cue questions: these are who, what, where, when, why, how?
- Writing an incident down provides a different perspective to thoughtful or spoken reflection

## Stage 3: Analysing the experience

At this stage in the process, you will be starting to take some steps back from your experience and attempting to treat it more objectively as a source of data to be broken down into its constituent parts. Here you start to ask the 'why' type of question as you explore the reasons behind what has happened. Now you are moving beyond the superficial elements of the first four key questions and it is here that you will draw conclusions from what you have recorded about the experience. As you progress through your course, and your academic career, you will increasingly be expected to reflect more deeply and with more insight, so that you achieve the key skills for the level at which you are studying. The skills of analysis are perhaps the first of these to be developed, as you move from the descriptive phases.

'Analysis' simply means to break things down into their constituent parts. For example, if you send a blood sample to a laboratory for

**○━ᴛ *Keywords***

**Analysis**
Breaking things down
and forming preliminary
conclusions

'analysis', what you get reported back are the proportions of its constituents. However, we expect analysis to go a little further than this, in terms of making some sort of judgement on the basis of this information. A laboratory report will, for instance, highlight where levels are within normal limits or fall outside of them. So, at this stage in our reflective processes, we will be expecting you to draw some preliminary conclusions as to the result of your analysis, such as 'What felt right about this experience and why?', or 'What actions caused this to go wrong, and why was this?'

When you first start reflective practice as part of your professional education, this is the stage at which you will probably stop initially. You will have begun to develop insight into the experiences you are exploring and to reach some conclusions about the part you played in them. This conscious awareness is crucial to the learning process, as we can use it to determine our future action. However, as you progress through your course, you will be expected to develop further through the levels of reflection (discussed in Chapter 3).

It is also at this stage that you may start to feel some discomfort about reflective practice as a strategy for learning. It may bring back memories of how you felt at the time or, alternatively, you may start to realise that what happened was a direct result of your part in the incident – what you did, how you acted, the choices you made. This is an inevitable part of using your own experiences to learn and a consequence of deliberately deciding to use these experiences as a source of learning. However, to some extent this is a very mature way of learning. We need to be willing to revisit our own actions, and we need to have some insight into ourselves. We also need to be able to accept responsibility for our own actions and the choices we make. For many students starting out on this path, this will be difficult, and that is why you will be asked to build reflective skills and strategies gradually. Part of this is to help you with your own self-development as you grow through your course. A professional who is expected to develop as an independent practitioner needs not only the knowledge and practical skills of their profession but also the insight and acceptance of their own actions that marks them as a responsible and safe practitioner. It is through the use of reflective practice, and developing the skills gradually and in a safe environment with the help of others, that you will add these skills to the 'kitbag' of tools that you use in your practice.

So, at this stage in the process, you may come to conclusions that you don't like very much or you feel reflect badly on you. However, this is not something to be anxious about provided that you remember, first, what the purpose of exploring the situation was and, second, what you hope to get out of it in terms of learning for the future.

---

**Key points** | Top tips

- Analysing means 'breaking experiences down and coming to some preliminary conclusions about them'
- You may begin to see the experience in a different way at this stage

---

## Stage 4: Interpreting the experience

During this stage you will develop a deeper understanding of the experience by exploring further the different parts of it. In the last stage you broke your experience down under different headings, such as 'What did I do and why?' or 'What did the other person do and why?' Here we want you to start thinking behind all these questions so that you understand a bit more about why things happened in the way that they did. You may choose to concentrate on just one or two of the features here and deal with them in detail. What you will end up with at this stage of the process is an *explanation*. This will enable you to move to the next phase of exploring alternatives, both interpreting the experience differently and seeing it in a different way.

Again, it is at this stage that you might find the process uncomfortable. Awkward questions may start popping into your head that you really don't want to think about. Or you may find that the incident dominates your thoughts when you are not deliberately reflecting on it. Don't worry! This is entirely natural and is part of the process of learning to reflect. As you become more skilled in the process you will be able to train yourself to limit your reflective activity to specific times that you set aside for it – maybe with other people or to compile a reflective journal for instance. At this stage in the process, though, try to focus on the future – think about the resolution of the process. The final two stages will bring you back to the top of the reflective cycle and will help you to move away from the experience as it was into perceptions of the experience that you haven't thought about and what action you need to take as a result. These final stages are the 'feel good' stages, where you can resolve a situation and decide to *deliberately* do something as a result of your explorations.

**Key points**  Top tips

- Interpretation involves considering your experiences in the light of other knowledge
- This will provide you with an explanation of the experience

## Stage 5: Exploring alternatives

At this stage you will be thinking about alternatives to the ways in which you have seen your experience initially. This is very challenging, in that it is asking you to look at different ways of understanding the experience to the way that you have described. Imagine looking at your experience as if you are not you at all! You will be trying to step out of your skin and see the whole experience from different viewpoints. To do this by yourself is quite difficult, so, initially, you will meet various different ways of reflecting, and be introduced to them in a variety of ways and in many settings – both academic and in the practice environment. You will also be encouraged to reflect with different types of people, from your colleagues to your practice supervisors; from other professional practitioners to your academic staff. From this you will build up a bank of both differing ways of reflecting and differing viewpoints from which to consider your experiences. The benefit of working within a multiprofessional environment is that we are always meeting others whose background provides them with different ways of seeing things and interpreting and explaining them. These enable us, in turn, to question our 'taken-for-granted' views and explorations of the world.

One way to understand this is to think of the way that the world appears if we put on different types of spectacles. Many of you will be lucky enough not to have to wear glasses at all; for others it is our every-day reality to put them on simply to get out of bed! Try to imagine how the world would look if we altered the types of glasses that we wear. For instance, if you smeared the lenses with grease, you would not have the clarity of view that you normally have, and everything would be out of focus. You would have to turn to your other senses, and your experience, to fill the gaps in the knowledge you use to make sense of what you are seeing. Another example is the way in which our perceptions change when it is dark – some things are hidden from us, we do not have the familiarity of colour and detail to help us and we have to rely on other ways of gaining information to help us to make decisions.

This is exactly what we do at this stage of the reflective process, in that we look for alternative ways of 'seeing' the experience. In a way, we have to 're-focus' our lenses in order to see things in a different way. We do this without thinking when we are dealing with the physical processes of trying to see in the dark. We automatically refocus our lenses to pick up on different cues that we don't need to use in daylight, and the ones that we normally use retreat to the background as they are redundant in those circumstances. We might even choose to use artificial aids, such as infra-red glasses, to enable us to see in a different way again.

At this stage in the reflective process, we will be consciously seeking ways of seeing the features of our experiences in a different way, for the purpose of learning more about them.

We may do this by ourselves, and use a reflective framework to help us, or we may choose to use others to reflect off, and use their perceptions to help us to see things from a different perspective.

The purpose of this stage, therefore, is to widen and deepen the experience for us by exploring other ways of 'seeing' what has occurred. Once we have done this, we can move to the final stage, which involves deciding how we can use what we have learned to identify what we need to do in the future.

---

**Key points**   Top tips

- Exploring alternatives is a challenging process as it asks us to step outside of our usual ways of seeing our experiences
- This stage enables us to explore alternative ways of perceiving things and working to those we would normally use

---

## Stage 6: Framing action

Arising from the previous stage will be several different possibilities for action that you might take. It is important here to make sure that you focus on *your* activity rather than expecting others to act for you or change themselves. This is *your* reflective learning and thus you only have responsibility for yourself – others hold their own responsibilities and make their own choices. While it may be comforting to propose courses of action for others that will make our lives easier, in reality motivation for change inevitably comes from within oneself. What we would like to see someone else do is not necessarily the right course of action for them, nor one that they would choose. Also, it will not necessarily alter the action or consequences for you in the end.

How often have you said of a partner, or a friend 'If only they would do what I told them to, it would all be so much simpler!' Unfortunately, life isn't like that.

So, the focus for framing action is on things that you can do that are within your control.

Of course, if you are helping another person to reflect, perhaps in clinical supervision or in a reflective activity, then your role will be to enable them to see their own alternatives and you may be able to suggest courses of action that they themselves haven't seen. As a result you may also shift your perspective and decide to change your own ways of dealing with something.

### The differences between reflective processes and reflective practice

Up to the end of this stage, what we have done is explore reflective processes, rather than necessarily reflective practice. By this we mean that we have not moved into the last element of reflective practice, which is to actually take the action that we have decided on.

At the end of the last stage, we were still operating in the realms of theoretical activity: we were talking about possibilities and what we might do. This could be, for instance, what we would do if the situation occurred again. Or it may be that we need to go to the library and get more information to add to the knowledge that underpinned how we dealt with the incident. Another possibility is that we decide we need to go and talk to someone else who is able to influence a situation that we are in. So, no action has been taken but the different courses of action have been explored.

It is important at this stage to consider not only what you might do but also the possible consequences of any course of action that you might take. In this way, a decision not to take action can be a deliberate choice, and in many ways is action! It differs from inactivity before reflection on the event because you have now thought through all aspects of the incident and consciously decided that overt action is not needed. You will, however, have a deeper understanding of the event and, perhaps more importantly, an understanding and overt acknowledgement of what you have learned about the experience.

Planning action has several features. First of all, the alternatives that you select from need to be possible in terms of:

- The scope of what you are trying to achieve

- The outcome you are trying to achieve

- The amount that you will need to rely on the help of other people

- The barriers you may encounter
- The resources you may need to carry them out.

Second, you need to be capable of carrying out the action.
You will need to think about:

- The time it will take
- Having access to relevant people
- Your own knowledge, skills and experiences
- Your motivation to carry out the action.

Finally, you will need to think about the consequences of any action that you might be considering, in terms of:

- Yourself
- Your patients/clients
- Your colleagues
- Your mentor/supervisor
- Other professional work colleagues
- Academic staff
- Your workplace
- Your role as a student
- Working within the code of professional conduct.

This may seem like a long list, and rather daunting at first. However, most of the time you will not need to consider all these aspects, and the list is here simply for you to think about when framing and planning any action. But sometimes we do omit to think about the consequences of the things that we do, and often this results in the unexpected coming at us. Hence, a cornerstone of professional practice is the ability to think through alternative courses of action in terms of the anticipated consequences for all concerned.

Once you have decided on the action that you will take from all of the possible alternatives, you are ready to carry it out.

**Key points** *Top tips*

- Framing action enables us to consider our future actions arising from the incident and its analysis
- The reflective processes end at this stage
- Reflective practice differs from reflective processes in that we turn thoughtful and possible activity into action

## Taking action

As the final phase of reflective practice, this is where you will carry out the action that you have decided upon. In many ways, this can be the easiest part of being a reflective practitioner – but in some ways it can be the hardest! This will depend of course on what it is that you have to do. It is here that you will move from the realms of the possible and probable into the real world. For instance, going to the library to research a topic to increase your knowledge is unlikely to be stressful. But other courses of action, especially where they involve confronting others or doing things that you find challenging or difficult and involve changes to your usual patterns of behaviour, will inevitably involve some anxiety or stress. This is entirely natural, and the way to manage it is to think about all the possible results of your action and plan for them in advance.

Factors you might like to consider are:

- **What you want to achieve as a result of your action.** This is where you will have ended the last stage of the reflective processes, so you should now have an idea of what your goals are in taking action. It is worth trying to write this concisely as a single sentence so that you have it clearly fixed in your mind. This also helps you to focus on the main purpose of taking action and to be single-minded in achieving your goal.

- **How you will do it.** Again, thinking through the possibilities of how you will take action helps you feel in control of the situation. You might like to plan the overall strategy that you will adopt, including:

- **When you will do it.** We have all heard the wisdom of 'sleeping on a problem'. It is often worth waiting before carrying out our decisions so that we can put some emotional distance between ourselves and the incident. However, just as pertinent is the need to resolve issues, so a happy medium between the two needs to be achieved. Perhaps the most important factor in terms of taking action is that it is your choice and under your control. Do you remember the times in the past that another person has caught you on the wrong foot by asking to talk to you about something that you weren't expecting at the time? For instance, were you ever called to see a teacher at school, or a supervisor at work, and you didn't know what it was about?

- **Where you will do it**

- **Who will be part of the action.**

## The importance of planning

There is an old adage 'to fail to plan is to plan to fail', and this is most appropriate in many aspects of student life. For instance, if you don't ensure that you understand what you are being asked to do in your assignments and plan your research and writing time in order to submit on time, and if you don't plan your revision strategies for exams, you are more likely to fail than if you do. In fact, omitting to plan is setting yourself up to fail. Students who pass all the elements of their course haven't done so by accident, they have planned to pass.

Similarly, when taking action as a result of our reflective activity, we can plan to be successful by thinking through all possible elements of the action that are within our control, to reduce the possibility of things going wrong.

One way of thinking about this is to recall other instances when you have decided to do something similar and remember the sense of relief and satisfaction that you felt once you had successfully resolved the issue. For instance, how many of us have dreaded returning goods to shops for fear of encountering aggressive shop assistants or being unable to achieve what we wanted from the interaction? Yet, with forethought and careful planning, knowing our rights in the circumstances and using good interpersonal skills, it is possible for both parties to achieve what they want without any problems. And the relief and positive feelings that result enable us to reflect on that experience as a learning opportunity, leading to less stress the next time a similar thing occurs. The combination of these successful encounters and the building up of cognitive skills as a result help to reduce the feelings of stress that we experience in other situations where we are worried about taking the action we need to. On the other hand, we are always likely to feel uncomfortable about not seeing things through to a conclusion, or taking the actions that we need to, as we are not experiencing closure of the incident or of the reflective cycle.

## *Reflective activity*

### Why do you do what you do?

Think back to the last time that you successfully tackled an issue you were anxious about. Reflect over the stages of what happened and what you did. What were the things that you did that made the incident successful? What from these would you use again in similar circumstances? How did resolving this incident make you feel? Did you find that after it was resolved the incident held less importance or significance for you?

Now think of an incident where you did not follow through on the course of action that you had decided was needed. Why did you decide not to act? How satisfied are you with the outcome of what happened? Do you find that you still think about the incident in a negative way? What do you think about it now? Is it still unfinished business?

No-one will claim that it is easy to take action to resolve situations that you have found difficult. But the rewards of doing so are many. Not least is the fact that you will be developing strategies for working in an environment that, by necessity, has to involve interactions between other people. But unresolved situations can cause stress, as we constantly think about what we did, or didn't do. They prevent us from achieving the things that we want to do because they take up our mental energy. Sometimes we just have to 'bite the bullet' and do something in order to get it out of the way, so that we can direct our energy into things that are more creative and positive.

Of course, if we do take the action as planned, we have created a new experience for ourselves, which in turn may be the focus of reflective activity. This is how the reflective cycle turns into the reflective spiral that we saw in Figure 1.3, earlier in the chapter.

### Key points | Top tips

- Taking action involves moving from the possible and probable into the real world
- It involves making decisions about what you will do and when, where and how you will do it
- It involves considering the roles of other people in your action
- Planning your action is more likely to result in success
- Failing to plan is planning to fail

## Identifying your role as a student in the clinical environment

When you enter the clinical environment to gain experience from practice, it is important to remember the primary reasons for you being there. These are:

- To learn from the experiences available
- To develop your competence in the practical aspects of your profession
- To acquire the professional attributes of a practitioner.

Essentially, these come down to one thing – to learn. However, you will be entering a working environment whose primary purpose is to deliver care to patients. A supplementary role for those working there is to support you as a student. Their priorities will revolve around patient care, and your needs will be subsumed below this. Therefore, the main person to look out for your needs is you! It is important to remember that, while you will get a great deal of help from other people, you are the only one who can ensure that you are gaining the experience that you need in order to achieve your learning outcomes. Using strategies for reflective practice will help you to do this in a conscious and planned way.

Students of health-care professions come from a wide range of backgrounds and life experiences. Many students now enter professional education as mature students, having already gained experience in a health-care support worker role to qualified staff. For these students, entering the clinical environment will not be as unfamiliar as for those students who are starting their courses straight from school or with little work experience. However, it is important to remember that everyone is an individual who already has life experiences that will stand them in good stead for their course. While mature students may envy the academic skills of students who have studied more recently, those with less (or no!) clinical experience may be considerably in awe of those who have earned a place on the course as a result of years of practical experience. It is important to remember that all students on a course are there to achieve competency in all areas of practice that will enable them to gain a professional qualification. All students enter the course having been selected because they have a profile of attributes, combining academic qualifications, a potential to achieve these, practical experience and the appropriate attitudes and values for health-care professions. These profiles are different for all students, providing a wealth of experiences and qualities that can be used as a resource for supporting and learning from each other.

One of these will be your own attitude towards learning, and your willingness to be open to new experiences, to put yourself in unfamiliar situations and learn from them. However much previous clinical experience you have, there is always more that can be learned. One of the key skills that you will need to develop as early as possible is to recognise and use learning opportunities in the clinical environment. These are explored in more detail in Chapter 4.

---

**Key points**   Top tips

- Your primary purpose in the clinical environment is to learn from the experiences available
- We can use these to build on our previous experiences
- It is important to recognise learning opportunities in the clinical environment

---

## Conclusions

In this chapter we have introduced you to the features of reflective practice so that you have a basic understanding to carry you through to the rest of the book. Especially important is becoming familiar with the stages of the ERA cycle through which reflective practice occurs. These stages, and the processes within them, are the key to your development as a reflective practitioner. The rest of the book develops each of the aspects that you have met in this chapter to help you acquire the skills and attributes of reflective practice by showing you how to do it.

---

*RRRRR***Rapid recap**

Check your progress so far by working through each of the following questions.

1. What is the ERA cycle of reflective practice?
2. What are Schön's two types of reflection?
3. What is the difference between the reflective processes and reflective practice?
4. What are the stages in the reflective processes?
5. What is meant by the term 'critical incident'?

If you have difficulty with more than one of the questions, read through the section again to refresh your understanding before moving on.

---

## References

Atkins, S. and Murphy, K. (1993) Reflection: a review of the literature. *Journal of Advanced Nursing*, **18** , 1188–1192.

CancerWeb Dictionary (2000) CancerNet database www.meb.uni_bonn.de/cancer.gov/index.

Dewey, J. (1938) *Experience and Education*. Macmillan, New York.

Flanagan, J. (1954) The Critical Incident Technique. *Psychological Bulletin*, **51**, 327–358.

Goodman, J. (1984) Reflection and teacher education: a case study and theoretical analysis. *Interchange*, **15**, 9–26.

Kolb, D. (1984) *Experiential Learning as the Science of Learning and Development*. Prentice Hall, Englewood Cliffs, NJ.

Rolfe, G., Freshwater, D. and Jasper, M. (2001) *Critical Reflection for Nursing and the Helping Professions: A user's guide*. Palgrave, Basingstoke.

Schön, D. (1983) *The Reflective Practitioner: How professionals think in action*. Temple Smith, London.

Webster's 3rd New International Dictionary (2000) Merriam-Webster, New York.

Wordnet 1.6 (1997) www.cogsci.princeton.edn/.

# 2

# Knowing ourselves

## Learning outcomes

By the end of this chapter you should be able to:

- Acknowledge your strengths and weaknesses and recognise how these can be built on for the future
- Explore the way you respond to challenges and acknowledge this as a way of managing strange situations
- Identify your beliefs and values as a professional practitioner
- Understand your learning style and how this influences the way in which you learn
- Identify your attitudes to writing and your writing style

Reflective practice takes its starting point from our experiences and assumes that we can learn from them for our future. Therefore the first place that we need to start in terms of our own reflective practice is by understanding ourselves. By knowing where we are starting from we can plan to build on our previous knowledge, understanding and skill as the foundations for our learning and development as professional practitioners. The purpose of this chapter is to lead you in recognising and exploring your previous experiences and own characteristics, attitudes and approaches to life so that you can actively use these in planning to succeed on your course. These can also be seen as the strategies that you use in your professional practice as you utilise them for learning and managing challenges. Hence, this chapter will get you reflecting on your own past experiences so far.

## Recognising our strengths and weaknesses

How often have you sat down in the past and really thought about what you are good at? How often do we draw attention to what we consider to be our failings, without acknowledging our strengths? Yet, crucial to being able to act as a professional practitioner is an understanding of our skills and abilities and an awareness of where the limits of these lie.

One of the ways that we can do this is to use a SWOB analysis to look analytically at ourselves. This involves thinking deeply to identify Strengths and Weaknesses. After this you broaden out into identifying what Opportunities are available to you, and what the Barriers might be in using these to achieve your aims. Key cue questions can be used to help you reflect on these four elements.

# *Reflective activity*

**Use the grid to complete
your own SWOB analysis.**

SWOB analysis grid

| Strengths | Weaknesses |
|---|---|
|  |  |
| Opportunities | Barriers |
|  |  |

Start with identifying your strengths. Although you are doing this in your capacity as a health-care student, do not limit what you write to simply what you think is appropriate to this role. Try to incorporate elements of all aspects of your experience such as your family life, your previous jobs, your educational experiences and any leisure time activities and interests that you have. Go behind these to identify the skills and experiences, the knowledge and understanding that has resulted in you being the person that you are today. Some of the elements you might like to consider are:

● What are you good at?

● What about yourself are you happy with?

● How do you get on with other people?

● What approaches do you take to life?

● What have you achieved so far in your life – what does this tell you about your strengths?

● What experiences have you had that provide a foundation for your course?

When thinking about your weaknesses, the purpose is not to find fault or blame yourself for anything. Instead, you will be making an honest assessment of where you feel you have room for improvement. So, initially, list all the things you can think of, whether you think they are under your control or not. Some cue questions might be:

● What would I like to change about myself?

● What things have not been successful?

● What things have I not achieved that I wanted to by now?

● What disappointments have I had that affect the ways I think about the future?

When you come to the Opportunities section try to build on what you have already identified as your strengths. For instance, if you have written 'I am good at working to deadlines' think how this can be used within your course over the next few years. Other cue questions might be:

● What is available within the course to help me?

● Who can help me?

● What support do I have that will help me?

In identifying the Barriers to your success, you might reflect on what the weaknesses you have identified tell you about yourself. How might you put up your own obstacles to success simply through the ways that you approach life? In fact, these might then become opportunities for your own development and change in the future and you may decide to move them. For instance, you may have young children who have calls on your time and therefore see this as a barrier to having as much time for study as you would wish. In fact, we all have limitations on our time for one reason or another. Having to apportion your time in various ways makes you think about the most effective ways of using it. So, you may decide that you will set aside specific time during the day that you can use for studying, and set boundaries to this. This would have the added effect of training your children so that they realise you need time to yourself and are not always at their beck and call.

Using a structure for reflection like this provides us with new ways of looking at things. It is rare in everyday life to be able to consider what makes us the person we are. We tend to be so busy simply getting through the day that we take for granted who and what we are. The case study below presents Hayley's SWOB analysis as she started a course for a dual qualification as a Social Worker and Registered Nurse for People with Learning Disabilities.

# Case study

## Hayley's SWOB analysis

| Strengths | Weaknesses |
|---|---|
| I have had 5 years experience as a care worker in a residential home for young people with severe learning disabilities | I tend to think that everyone is as enthusiastic as me |
| I understand the challenges of working with people with communication problems | I am not very good at writing essays |
| I have good practical skills | I am not confident in my own abilities and tend to stay quiet |
| I am not afraid of hard work | I am reserved with new people |
| I am highly motivated and determined to succeed | I tend to retreat into the background in group situations |
| I am good at communicating with people | I am critical of myself and think I can't do things |
| I am very patient with other people | |
| I am an optimist – nothing much gets me down | |
| I value all people for who and what they are | |
| I tend not to be critical of others | |
| I have succeeded in getting three A levels as a mature student | |
| I put other people's needs before my own | |
| I have three children and manage a home as a single parent | |
| I sing in a choir | |

| Opportunities | Barriers |
|---|---|
| I have a place on the course, support from my employer and my salary | Balancing and managing my time so that I can fit in everything that I need to do |
| I can use my previous experiences within the course and build on these | Not having a computer at home and not having any IT skills |
| I can use the resources in college to build my academic skills, help me with my confidence building and assertiveness | Looking after the children |
| I can use my placements to build up my skills in different areas | Travelling to college and placements |
| I have the maturity to acknowledge my limitations and ask for help and support | Choir practice |
| | My lack of confidence in myself |
| | My lack of assertiveness |

The benefits in doing this at the start of a course is that we can actively and consciously use what we have found about ourselves in planning our strategies for the future. So the next step in this exercise is to form an action plan.

Part of the process of action planning is to be willing to think differently about something, and find ways of overcoming problems that you had not previously considered. In Hayley's case, for instance, she had always felt that her children's needs came first and that, as a result, she was less important. She had got into the habit of doing all the housework because it was easier than nagging at the children, and always spent Sunday evening doing the ironing in front of the television. However, she realised as a result of the SWOB analysis that there were ways in which she, the children, and the situation would have to change if she was to be able to find the time to study at home.

She sat down with the children and together they worked out ways that they could all take some responsibility around the house, starting with a rota for the washing up and putting away after meals. All three took responsibility for keeping their rooms tidy. However, after thinking about it, Hayley realised that it was her problem that she wanted the rooms tidy, and not theirs! So, a compromise was negotiated so that the rooms they shared, especially the living room, would be kept tidy, and the boys could live in their rooms as they pleased, provided it did not interfere with anyone else. They also devised a rota for sharing out the washing, ironing and cleaning the bathroom, agreeing to rotate this every week. Hayley had to teach the boys to iron effectively, and they learned basic skills for feeding themselves and cooking simple meals for the whole family.

Previously, Hayley could not have conceived of expecting her boys to take part in all the tasks that she felt were her responsibility as a mother. But, through the necessity of having to create more time in her busy life, she had to stand back and force herself to think about things in a different way. She realised that untidy bedrooms were not really that important – especially if she didn't go into them! She found very quickly that the boys would not go hungry if she did not have food on the table, and that in fact one of them was turning out to be a very good cook. She also realised that, while she needed to be more active as a housekeeper when the children were small, much of what she was doing she did out of habit, and she hadn't kept up with their growth and abilities. In providing them with the opportunities to take more responsibility in the house she was facilitating them into adulthood and preparing them for a time when they too would live independently or with their own partners.

Hayley had turned what could have been a huge barrier to success into positive opportunities for herself and her boys. Not only that, she found she had 6 hours per week extra study time – time that had previously simply disappeared into routine house work, which was still getting done but in a different way.

The necessity to find a solution to a problem, and using a potential barrier as a stimulus for changing her way of thinking, was also a positive learning experience for Hayley. It made her realise how she had got into the habit of thinking the ways she did and thought about things were the only ways. A willingness to put aside the things we take for granted, or to reconsider things that we think are fixed and beyond our control, are the first steps in enabling our own personal development. They will also help us move in different ways of experiencing our lives.

## *Reflective activity*

Work through all of the features that you identified in your SWOB analysis and formulate a plan of action from them.

First of all, plan to reinforce your strengths by making the most of your opportunities.

Next think about your weaknesses. Many of these you may think are outside your control. But, when you consider it, they are your weaknesses, not anyone else's, and therefore it is only you that can do anything about them! Recognising and taking responsibility for doing something about the things you don't like about yourself is a major step. Going a bit further and actually doing something about it is just one more! So, if you find yourself glossing over some of these, stop, consider why you are trying to avoid dealing with them and perhaps set yourself a challenge by tackling at least one.

Similarly, it is important to start making plans to tackle or overcome the barriers that you identified. As Hayley did, try to look at a problem in a different way to your normal perspective. If necessary, bounce the problem off another person to see whether they see it in a different way to you, or can propose a solution that you hadn't thought about.

The final step, of course, is to put the plan into action! And only you can decide to do that…

In completing this activity, you have taken the first steps in reflective practice. You have certainly completed the ERA reflective cycle, possibly several times if you have actually sorted out many of the issues that you had identified.

This illustrates that reflective practice is not simply confined to our professional practice. Using the techniques and strategies of reflective practice enables us to become more aware of the ways in which we live our lives and more open to the possibilities of alternatives and change.

Using reflection to identify our needs, and courses of action for the future makes it a very positive strategy. This section also illustrates that reflection need not simply focus on a single incident, nor remain in the realms of the past – using reflection to inform the future is its most significant and valuable feature.

> **Key points** | Top tips
>
> - Identifying our strengths helps us to value ourselves and build on these for the future
> - Identifying our weaknesses allows us to plan to remedy them
> - Identifying our opportunities ensures that we are aware of options available to us
> - Identifying the barriers in our lives helps us to take a fresh look at where we are and how to change

## Coping with challenges

Within your SWOB analysis it is likely that you drew attention to the ways in which you cope with challenges in your life. You may have identified these as both strengths and weaknesses. Look back on these now and consider whether you want to add more features in here.

Basically, just about anything that we do is a challenge, and we adopt very similar ways of tackling these, no matter what they are. On the whole, we manage these well, and as a result tend not to think of them as challenges at all – for instance, organising a birthday party or applying for a passport. The very fact that you have started your course means that you are successful in meeting the challenges of gaining the appropriate entry criteria, completing the application process successfully, surviving the selection process and turning up on the first day!

In considering events and experiences to be challenges though, we often focus only on the negative things that happen to us, or the things that go wrong. These occur because the usual ways that we cope with things have failed us on these occasions. They tend to stay in our mind for longer and as a result we may start to believe that we are not good at certain things or can't cope in certain situations. If we look at these events in a different way however, we are able to deal with them in the same way as we would when things (usually) work out the way we want them to. By understanding the ways in which we would normally approach a situation, and being aware of this, we can plan to use this in situations that we find difficult.

## Reflective activity

Think back to the last time that you organised a holiday.

**What did you do?**

Your approach to planning a holiday is probably typical of the ways in which you tackle most challenges that you know about. All of us will go about this in different ways but, on the whole, the strategies that we adopt enable us to succeed. In recognising these, and actively using them throughout your course, you are more likely to be successful.

Now, think about a challenge that took you by surprise – perhaps the washing machine broke down mid-cycle or the car engine started billowing steam while you were driving it.

**What did you do?**

Once we get over the initial shock of an unexpected challenge, we tend to use the same coping strategies as when we have time to forward plan. By analysing your responses to things that hit you out of the blue, you will see how you are likely to react to these sort of events in your clinical practice.

Health-care practice is characterised by the unexpected, and therefore you need to recognise the ways in which you deal with this. You will need to actively develop strategies that will enable you to function effectively in these situations. Clearly, your course and your supervisors in practice will help you. But there are many things that you can do for yourself through planning to recognise and deal with your own reactions. By drawing on the ways that you know you have dealt with challenges successfully in the past, you will begin to eradicate the behaviours that have prevented you from coping. For instance, panic reactions, running away and asking someone else to deal with things are not going to develop your own confidence and competence as a practitioner.

## Over to you

Actively recognising the ways in which you cope with challenges, and planning to change any behaviour that prevents you from dealing with them effectively is within your control. Next time something happens that you see as a challenge, take note of how you feel, think and react. Later, ask yourself what you did that was effective, and what was less so. Think about these reactions and try to use more of those that are effective and change the negative responses in the future.

Having focused on yourself as a person, we now turn to you as a practitioner.

## Knowing ourselves as practitioners

When we enter a profession we bring with us our own beliefs and values and the perceptions of it we have developed over the years. For some reason, we have chosen to enter this particular profession, and often we have only a vague understanding of why this is.

However, the type of practitioner we become is dependent upon these underpinning beliefs and values, and it is therefore worth taking some time to become aware of what they are.

### *Reflective activity*

#### Choosing a professional specialty

**What was it that attracted you to the health-care specialty that you have entered?**

Try to think about this in terms of:

- The type of service you provide
- The knowledge and skills you will develop
- The type of work you will be doing
- The types of patient you will be dealing with
- The relationships you will have with your patients
- The amount of professional autonomy and independence you will have
- The environments in which you will work
- The relationships you will have with other professional groups
- Your career prospects
- Your previous experiences of the profession.

The answers that you have given in this activity will have painted a picture of your chosen professional group. This may have changed as a result of your experiences so far on your course, as you enter the real world of the profession as opposed to the one you imagined before. It will continue to change as you move through your educational preparation and as you gain the 'hands-on' experience that turns you from an onlooker to a practitioner in your own right. Your views are also likely to change once you have qualified and start to try out and use your knowledge and skills in a professional capacity. You will also be taking

**⊶ᴛ** *Keywords*

**Accountable**
Being able to justify our
actions to others and take
responsibility for them

**Socialisation processes**
The interactions that we have
with others that enable us to
learn how to fit into different
social situations, e.g. learning
the rules of working in a
specific profession

on the responsibilities of providing a safe and competent service for
your patients, as well as being **accountable** for your own actions.

## Where do our beliefs and values come from?

As soon as we start to become social beings we begin to learn the
beliefs and values of our society. The **socialisation processes** that we
go through, from our early experiences at home, through our school
years, college and into adulthood, all provide us with ideas about what
is right and wrong, and what are acceptable attitudes and behaviour.
There are many influences on us as we grow and mature into adulthood,
and hence we absorb, unconsciously, the ways in which we view the
world. As a result, when we enter professional education, we bring
with us a preformed picture of the way the profession is. We also have
a picture of the person who is a professional. These influences may
come from:

- Previous personal experience of the profession
- Knowing someone in the profession
- Media influences – TV, newspapers, books, magazines,
  advertising material
- Careers information.

The pictures we have of our profession tend to be idealised and are not
really a representation of the 'real-life' experience of the profession as
it happens every day. Your views of the profession will be modified by
the 'insider' experiences, as opposed to those of an outsider looking in.
The influences that will help you in developing your beliefs and values
and gain a more realistic picture may come from:

- Your own fundamental beliefs and values, derived from the culture
  you have grown up in
- Your own personality, attitudes and approach to life
- Other professionals – practitioners, educators
- Codes of professional conduct
- Societal ethical and moral codes and values.

Much of the way in which you learn these, and take on the attributes
of your profession, will be through role modelling other practitioners.
Identifying role models and thinking about what it is that makes them
the type of professional practitioner you admire, is a useful way of
learning how to develop the characteristics of your professional group.
All the practitioners you meet during your course will have some sort
of impact on you. You will, probably quite unconsciously, select some
of these as role models because you admire and respect the ways in

which they conduct themselves as practitioners. On the other hand, you will identify some people as poor role models for you because their behaviour makes you feel uncomfortable in some way.

## *Reflective activity*

### What is a professional practitioner?

You can do this exercise either by yourself or with other people. Sometimes it is useful to work with others in this way, because they may see other things that you have not thought about and therefore you see a broader picture than one that you would have developed by yourself.

First of all, think about and list the characteristics of the type of person that you thought would be typical of a practitioner in your profession before you started your course. For instance, you might think about the way they look, or the way that they interact with other people. Have you a role model who, for instance, made you think about joining your profession? Or maybe you have seen portrayals on television of different kinds of health professional that gave you some ideas about how you think they work.

Now take some time to think about the attributes of a practitioner that you have already met and worked with that you admire. For instance:

- Initially, what was it that made them stand out for you?
- What is it about them that you want to be like?
- How do they interact and relate with patients?
- How do they interact and relate with other members of staff?
- How do they conduct themselves as a professional person? For instance, think about how they embody their code of professional conduct, how they maintain the confidentiality, respect and dignity for their patients
- How do they present themselves in terms of their speech, dress and ways of working?
- How knowledgeable are they about their practice?

Now think about someone who you do not admire, who perhaps has done something that stands out in your mind and makes you think that you do not want to be like them. Discuss their characteristics with a colleague, or note them down.

- What was it that they did that made you remember them?
- Why did you decide that you did not want to be like that?
- What standards can you use to assess their behaviour (e.g. the code of professional conduct, other professional standards, everyday expectations of the ways in which people deserve to be treated)

By now you will be building up a picture of the type of practitioner you want to become and also forming some ideas of the type that you don't want to be like. Engaging in reflective practice, using your clinical experiences, will help you recognise your own developing professional persona, and you will be able to constantly check that you are comfortable with the image you see emerging.

Throughout your course you will be challenged constantly by encountering practice that makes you feel uncomfortable. This might be because you are unhappy with the way that a person behaves, or it might be that you witness episodes of care that do not reach a safe standard. These episodes, while disappointing, because they dispel our illusions about professional practice, can also serve a useful purpose in helping us to recognise, and reinforce, our own underpinning professional values and beliefs.

By sharing your reflections on your experiences in health care you will be developing an understanding of your own values, beliefs and ideas about your chosen profession. You will also come to understand how other people can operate with a different set of ideas that, although not the same as yours, provides them with an effective starting point for their own practice. Despite the effects of education and experience in practice, we all develop our own unique set of beliefs and values that inform the ways in which we practise. Most of these, for most people, fall within parameters that are considered acceptable. One of the purposes of allocating you to supervisors in practice is to help you to develop these acceptable beliefs and values, which will designate you as a person worthy of practising independently.

However, if people display unacceptable behaviour, either attitudinally or through their treatment of other people, they will be sanctioned.

As a student this may mean that your supervisors and lecturers help you to develop more appropriate ways of conducting yourself, or help you to see things in the way that is acceptable to your profession. In order to be accepted on to the professional register in some professions, your lecturers have to sign a declaration of 'good character'. Without this, even if you have successfully passed all of your course components, you will be unable to register as a practitioner. This may happen, for instance, if you commit an illegal act, such as stealing from patients, but can also occur if others do not approve of the way in which you act and can present a case against you. When you qualify, you can be removed from the register if it is proved that you have contravened the code of professional conduct. This, of course, is the most serious penalty that can be imposed on you. However, your employer can dismiss you from your job for misconduct as well, and all employers have disciplinary processes that can be used to draw your attention to unacceptable behaviour.

In this section you will have developed a deeper understanding of your own beliefs about your profession and the people who work

## *Reflective activity*

### Myself as a practitioner

This is a challenging exercise as it asks you to really think about your own beliefs and values, which are contributing to the type of practitioner you will become. Try to complete the sentences below. This is a useful exercise to do with other people, and the trick here is to not look down the list of questions but to take them one by one.

1.  As a student in the clinical environment, I like to be called......... because.........
2.  My practice experience so far includes.........
3.  I want to be a......... practitioner because.........
4.  I believe I will be a good practitioner because.........
5.  My philosophy of practice is.........
6.  I believe that the most important part of my job is.........
7.  I believe that good practitioners have the characteristics of.........
8.  My relationship to my patient is as a.........
9.  I carry out this relationship by.........
10. My status in regard to my patient is.........
11. The environment in which I am most effective in my job is.........
12. The environment in which I would like to do my job is.........
13. My definition of care is.........
14. The part I play in other people's care is.........
15. I achieve this by.........
16. I understand holistic care to mean.........
17. In my practice I achieve this by.........
18. Some of my strengths as a practitioner are.........
19. Some of my weaknesses are.........
20. To become more effective as a practitioner I have to work on:
    a. Understanding my philosophy of practice
    b. Skills such as.........
    c. My theoretical approach
    d. My personal growth
    e. Other things such as.........
21. The things that I need to learn in order for me to do this are.........
22. I will achieve this by.........

Now spend a few minutes reviewing what you have learnt from this exercise in terms of:

● Your own beliefs and values
● Other people's beliefs and values (if you have done this with others)
● How useful this has been as an exercise in helping you to identify your guiding principles
● Its usefulness as a reflective strategy
● What action you need to take as a result of the things you have learnt

in it, and your own beliefs and values that underpin your role as a practitioner in your field. It is worth revisiting these at different stages in your course and comparing what you think then with what your initial impressions were. It will be interesting to see whether your views and perceptions change as you progress through your course. It is also useful to ask yourself why this might be and whether you need to take stock of where you are at the time and re-think the ways in which you approach your practice.

**Key points** Top tips

- We all work as professionals from a distinct and individual values base
- Many of these values come from our previous experiences of the profession
- Many of these will come from our experiences of working with others
- Recognising our values is crucial to understanding who we are as practitioners and how we practise

## Identifying your learning style

Just as we all have different personalities, so we all have preferences about the ways that we learn. Mostly these are unconscious: we don't usually deliberately choose the types of activity that suit us because we are, more often than not, unaware that some methods suit us and some don't. The purpose of this section is to help you to explore your past experiences of learning from a variety of situations in order to enable you to identify your **learning style** and recognise how this affects the way that you plan.

Most of the learning that we are aware of takes place in a formal learning situation where teaching and learning methods are not chosen by us but are imposed by others such as teachers, mentors and lecturers. Many of us find learning in these formal situations a challenge, and often one that we choose not to engage in once we leave school or college. Sometimes we even label ourselves as failures because we don't seem to be able to learn in the way others want us to, and we blame ourselves for not being able to cope with the material that is thrown at us.

However, being unable to learn in these situations is not necessarily a result of not being capable of doing the work, or learning the skill. It may be down to the teaching and learning approach that is used. It may simply be that you don't learn in that way! For instance, many people find it difficult to start with a theory and then apply it to practice. How many times have you said 'I don't know what you are talking about, just show me.' This often happens when we are dealing with practical skills that you need to understand the theoretical basis for. For instance, some people are quite comfortable with learning the wiring diagram of a plug and then going and practising the skills. Others, however, want to be shown how to do it and then to go back to the theory afterwards. In formal learning situations, we tend to be faced with the theory of something first, and only once we have mastered this are we allowed to go and practise. If you find it difficult to learn in this way, if you are one of the people who need to 'see' something before they can understand, the formal methods of learning that are used may be preventing you from learning, or at least they may be contributing to any problems you may have.

In adult learning situations, such as university, evening classes or even college courses that attract post-school students, it is likely that you will meet a variety of teaching and learning methods. They are designed to help everyone, at some stage, to select the methods that are most likely to help them to learn effectively in a way that suits them.

Having an awareness of the ways in which we learn best, the ways that we would choose to learn if we were left to ourselves, helps us to select from these methods to maximise our opportunities.

## Over to you

Think back over your learning experiences so far in your life. These will include both formal educational experiences, and also those less formal, where you have perhaps learned things at home, in your workplace, or in your leisure time.

Make a list of the types of activity that you have used, and find an example that you have used each for.

Now, for each one, write down what you liked about it and what you didn't, whether it involved some activity on your part or whether it was a largely passive technique.

Finally, think about how effective it was for you in helping you to learn, and whether you felt any emotional response when using it, such as excitement, frustration or anxiety. Give it a score out of 10 for how comfortable you felt in using it over all.

What you have done here is to start to identify the types of situation that suit you best and those that you feel most comfortable with.

The basis of this is that we all have a 'preferred learning style'. What this means is that the basic underlying features of our personality make some ways of learning more suitable for us as an individual than others.

## How to identify your learning style

The questionnaire below (Table 2.1) is designed to find out your preferred learning style(s). Over the years you have probably developed learning habits that help you benefit more from some experiences than from others. Since you are probably unaware of this, this questionnaire will help you to pinpoint your learning preferences so that you are in a better position to select learning experiences that suit your style. It was first designed by David Kolb in 1970 (Kolb 1984).

There is no time limit to this questionnaire, but it will probably take about 10–15 minutes. There are no right or wrong answers. Look at the four statements in each row and decide how they refer to you. Allocate four marks to the statement nearest to you, three to the second, two to the third and one to the statement least like you.

**Table 2.1  The learning style inventory  (Kolb 1984)**

| | a | b | c | d |
|---|---|---|---|---|
| **1** | I like to get involved | I like to take my time before acting | I am particular about what I like | I like things to be useful |
| **2** | I like to try things out | I like to analyse things and break them down into parts | I am open to new experiences | I like to look at all sides of issues |
| **3** | I like to watch | I like to follow my feelings | I like to be doing things | I like to think about things |
| **4** | I accept people and situations the way they are | I like to be aware of what is around me | I like to evaluate | I like to take risks |
| **5** | I have gut feelings and hunches | I have a lot of questions | I am logical | I am hard working and get things done |
| **6** | I like concrete things I can see, feel, touch and smell | I like to be active | I like to observe | I like ideas and theories |
| **7** | I prefer learning in the here and now | I like to consider and reflect about them | I tend to think about the future | I like to see the results of my work |
| **8** | I have to try things out for myself | I rely on my own ideas | I rely on my own observations | I rely on my own feelings |
| **9** | I am quiet and reserved | I am energetic and enthusiastic | I tend to reason things out | I am responsible about things |

Use the grid in Table 2.2 to summarise your score on the Learning Style inventory and fill in your total score for each column in the spaces below.

| Table 2.2 **Scoring grid for learning styles inventory** | | | |
|---|---|---|---|
| **CE Concrete experience** | **RO Reflective observation** | **AC Abstract conceptualisation** | **AE Active experimentation** |
| 1a | 1b | 2b | 2a |
| 2c | 2d | 3d | 3c |
| 3b | 3a | 4c | 6b |
| 4a | 6c | 6d | 7d |
| 8d | 8c | 8b | 8a |
| 9b | 9a | 9c | 9d |
| **Total** | **Total** | **Total** | **Total** |

Only put down the 'marks' asked for. You will notice that the marks for 1c and 1d are not asked. This is intended to stop 'patterning' and is not a mistake.

Now use the scores you have from the four columns in the following way.
First, subtract your RO score from your AE score.
Second, subtract your CE score from your AC score.
Plot the resulting figures on the two axes in Figure 2.1.

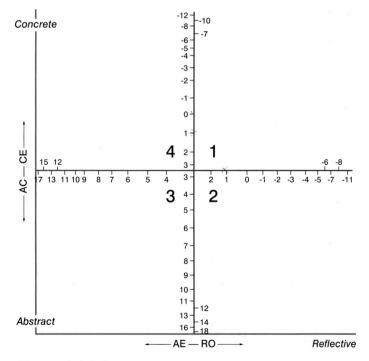

**Figure 2.1** *Axis diagram*

The four scores you originally arrived at can be plotted on to Figure 2.2 and joined up to produce your 'kite'.

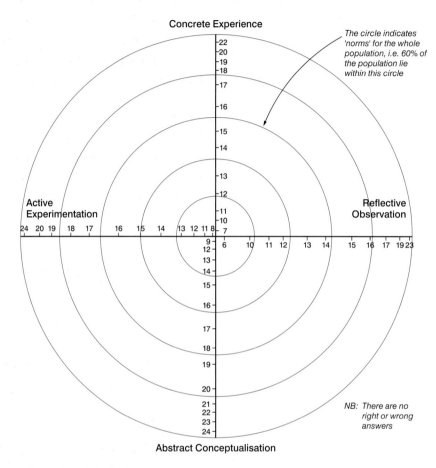

**Figure 2.2** *Kite diagram*

The shape of your kite gives you a profile of your learning style and the ways in which you are likely to learn best. Kolb suggests that we collect and use our experiences in one of two ways:

- We can gather experiences first hand by 'living the experience' – Kolb calls this **concrete experience** (CE)
- We can gather experience second-hand by being told about or reading about it – Kolb calls this **abstract conceptualisation** (AC)

The CE–AC axis is often called the Grasping Line.

We transform our experiences into knowledge again in one of two ways:

- We reflect on the experiences received in a considered and impartial manner. Kolb refers to this as **reflective observation** (RO)
- We are more concerned with seeking out the practical applications. Kolb calls this **active experimentation** (AE)

The RO–AE axis is often referred to as the Transforming Line.

## Preferred learning quadrant

The combination of scores on the kite indicates your preferred learning style. We all learn to grasp experiences and transform them into knowledge in all four ways. Combinations of preferred ways of grasping and transforming knowledge give rise to the preferred learning style which correspond to the quadrants in Figure 2.3.

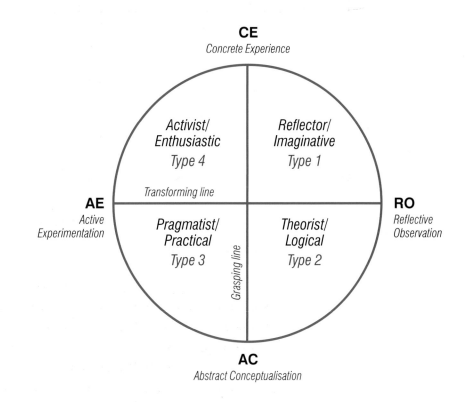

**Figure 2.3** *Preferred learning styles quadrant*

No-one learns exclusively in just one style, but we all tend to fall mostly under the one descriptor and 'borrow' characteristics from the others. McCarthy (cited by Kolb 1984) summarises the four types of learner in Table 2.3.

---

### Table 2.3 Types of learner (adapted from Kolb 1984)

**Type four learner:** Activist/Enthusiastic

Integrates experience and application

Seeks hidden possibilities, excitement

Needs to know what can be done with things

Learns by trial and error, self-discovery

Seeks influence and solidarity

Enriches reality

Perceives information concretely and processes it actively

Is adaptable to change and relishes it, likes variety and excels in situations calling for flexibility

Tends to take risks, at ease with people, sometimes seen as pushy

Often reaches conclusions in the absence of logical justification

Functions by acting and testing experience

**Strengths:** Action, carrying out plans

**Goals:** To make things happen, to bring action to concepts

**Favourite question:** What if?

**Type one learner:** Reflector/Imaginative

Integrates experience with the 'self'

Seeks meaning, clarity and integrity

Needs to be personally involved

Seeks commitment

Learns by listening and sharing ideas

Values insight, thinking, works for harmony

Absorbs reality

Perceives information concretely and processes it reflectively

Interested in people and culture

Divergent thinkers who believe in their own experience and excel in viewing concrete situations from many perspectives

Model themselves on those they respect

**Strengths:** Innovations and imagination. They are ideas people. They function through social integration and values clarification

**Goals:** Self-involvement in important issues, bringing unity to diversity

**Favourite question:** Why?

**Type three learner:** Pragmatist/Practical

Practises and personalises

Seeks usability, utility, solvency, results

Needs to know how things work

Learns by testing theories in ways that seem most sensible

Values strategic thinking, is skills-oriented

Edits reality

Perceives information abstractly and processes it actively

Uses factual data to build designed concepts, needs hands-on experiences, enjoys solving problems, resents being given answers

Restricts judgement to concrete things, has limited tolerance for 'fuzzy' ideas

Need to know how things they are asked to do will help in real life

Functions through inferences drawn from their bodies

They are decision makers

**Strengths:** Practical application of ideas

**Goals:** To bring their view of the present into line with future security

**Favourite question:** How does this work?

**Type two learner:** Theorist/Logical

Forms theories and concepts

Seeks facts and continuity

Needs to know what the experts think

Seeks goals attainment and personal effectiveness

Learns by thinking through ideas

Values sequential thinking, needs details

Forms reality

Perceives information and collects data

Thorough and industrious, re-examines facts if situations are perplexing

Enjoys traditional classrooms

Schools are designed for these learners

Functions by thinking things through and adapting to experts

**Strengths:** Creating concepts and models

**Goals:** Self-satisfaction and intellectual recognition

**Favourite question:** What?

There are many ways in which we can plan to work with our learning style once we have recognised it. At the very least it helps us to understand why each person seems to learn better from different teaching and learning methods and why we should try to incorporate a range of methods into a course for students. While we all learn to adapt to the methods that we need to use, some will find that they prefer one over another. Hence the reason that some people naturally seem to take to reflective processes and practices as learning strategies, where others struggle to grasp even the fundamentals and find it more challenging.

Often we have no choice in the ways in which we learn: for instance, lectures, seminars and group work, and individual tutorials are always likely to be a feature of formal educational settings. However, there are times, particularly when you are working independently in clinical placements or have private study time, that you can choose the learning methods you use. This is where the predominance of your preferred style of learning is likely to come to the fore, and you will select methods that you feel most comfortable with, or even enjoy! Table 2.4 identifies the types of learning activity that people with each learning style are likely to gain the most from – and conversely, the type of activity least likely to engage them.

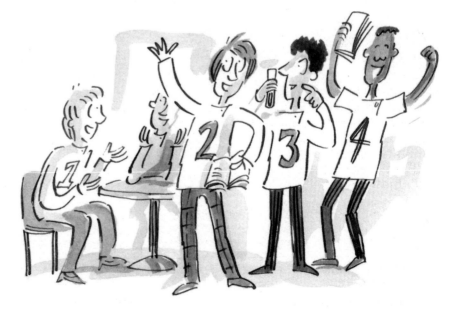

*Recognising which type of learner you are will help with your future development*

## Table 2.4 Learning activities and learning styles

| | Type 4:<br>Activist/enthusiastic | Type 1:<br>Reflector/Imaginative | Type 3:<br>Pragmatist/practical | Type 2:<br>Theorist/logical |
|---|---|---|---|---|
| **Learns best from activities where:** | There are new experiences, problems or opportunities<br><br>Short 'here and now' activities are used, e.g. role play<br><br>There is excitement, drama or crisis and a range of diverse activities to tackle<br><br>They have the limelight, e.g. chairing meetings, leading discussions<br><br>There is opportunity to generate ideas without the constraint of policy, structure or feasibility<br><br>They are thrown in at the deep end with a task they think is difficult<br><br>They are involved with other people<br><br>It is appropriate to have a go | They are encouraged to watch, think and chew over activities<br><br>They can stand back from events and listen and observe<br><br>They can think before acting<br><br>They can thoroughly research the problem<br><br>They have the opportunity to review what has been learned<br><br>They are asked to produce carefully considered analyses and reports<br><br>They are helped to exchange ideas with other people without danger<br><br>They can reach a decision in their own time without tight deadlines | There is an obvious link between the theory and the problem on the job<br><br>They are shown techniques with obvious practical advantages<br><br>They can try out and practise techniques with feedback from a credible expert<br><br>They are exposed to a model they can emulate<br><br>They are given techniques currently applicable to their job<br><br>They are given immediate opportunity to implement what is learned<br><br>There is validity in the learning activity, i.e. real problems<br><br>They can concentrate on practical issues | What is being offered is part of a system, model, concept or theory<br><br>They can explore the associations between ideas<br><br>They can question and probe the basic assumptions or logic<br><br>They are intellectually stretched<br><br>They are in structured situations with a clear purpose<br><br>They can listen to ideas that emphasise rationality and are well argued<br><br>They can analyse and generalise the reasons for success or failure<br><br>They are offered interesting ideas even though they are not immediately relevant<br><br>They are required to understand and participate in complex situations |
| **Learns least from activities where:** | Learning involves a passive role<br><br>They need to stand back and not be involved<br><br>They are required to deal with a lot of 'messy' data<br><br>They are involved in solitary work<br><br>Theoretical statements are used<br><br>The same activity is repeated over and over again<br><br>There are precise instructions to follow with little room for manoeuvre<br><br>They are asked to do a thorough job and attend to detail | They are forced into the limelight<br><br>They are forced into situations that require action without planning<br><br>They are thrown into something without warning<br><br>They are given insufficient data on which to base a conclusion<br><br>They are given cut and dried instructions on how things should be done<br><br>In the interest of expediency, they have to make short cuts | There is no context or apparent purpose<br><br>Emotions and feelings are emphasised<br><br>They are involved in unstructured activities where ambiguity and uncertainty are high<br><br>They are asked to decide without a basis in policy, principle or concept<br><br>Learning is superficial<br><br>They doubt that the subject matter is methodologically sound<br><br>They find the subject matter shallow or gimmicky<br><br>They feel out of tune with the other participants | The learning is not related to an immediate need<br><br>Organisers of the learning seem distant from reality<br><br>There is no practice or guidelines on how to do the task<br><br>They feel that people are going round in circles and not getting anywhere fast enough<br><br>There are political, managerial or personal obstacles to implementation<br><br>They cannot see sufficient reward from the learning activity. |

**Over to you**

You might like to spend some time now considering the implications for yourself of identifying your preferred learning style and how you can plan to use that in your learning.

**Key points** ~~Top tips~~

- Recognising our preferred learning style is a short cut way to making the most of our learning experiences
- We can plan to use learning strategies that tie in with our preferred learning style
- As reflective learning from experience is self-dependent, we have choice and control over what strategies we use

## Identifying your writing style

During your course you are going to be doing a lot of writing. This will take many forms and have different purposes. Underpinning these is the basic approach you take to writing, arising from your learning style and personality. It is worth thinking more about this because in understanding how we write we can make choices about the ways we use writing as a learning strategy in itself.

First of all, though, we'd like to explore where our ideas about writing come from in the first place. As with most of our ideas, our perceptions, attitudes and feelings about writing come from the experiences we have had in doing it. Let's face it, we write every day, and for most of us the physical and psychological acts of writing have become second nature. We may, for instance, unhesitatingly write a shopping list or a note to a friend. But there are other kinds of writing that evoke emotional responses, such as writing business letters, constructing an essay or sitting an examination.

> ## Reflective activity
>
> Think back over the past 10 years and on the left hand side of your page write a list of the different types of writing that you have done in this time, leaving a few lines between each one.
>
> On the other side of the page, for each type of writing that you listed, answer the following questions:
>
> 1. What was the purpose of writing?
> 2. Who were you writing for?
> 3. Who set the rules for that type of writing?
> 4. What part of it did you control and what components were controlled by others?

Our awareness of the different writing styles, dictated by the 'rules' for that particular style, enables us to select the one most appropriate to why we are writing. Look back over your list. How many of these were under the control of others or written according to 'rules' or conventions that you have learned in the past? The list that I came up with was:

- Writing essays
- Writing research reports
- Records of patient/client care and interaction
- Recording observations
- Giving written feedback to students
- Writing for publication
- Writing a job application
- Constructing a CV
- Writing for my professional portfolio
- Writing for my journal
- Sending memos and e-mails
- Letters – for work, to friends, for references
- Sending Christmas and birthday cards

This list is not exhaustive, but many of these have certain 'rules' that define what is supposed to be acceptable in that type of written communication. While there is room for individual style within these, we learn the difference, for instance, between writing a letter to a friend and writing a letter of complaint, or a job application. On the whole, these rules serve positive purposes in enabling us to operate within the various roles that we lead in our lives. By knowing what is expected and what is not, we can operate within a safety zone, where we present the public side of ourselves to others.

But, we also write for ourselves, probably every day. You might not have thought about things like shopping lists, notes to your family, notes from the reading that you do, your diary (if you keep one), even notes to the milkman! But, when you think about it, these are all instances of writing, and probably ones that we are so comfortable with that we don't think of them as writing at all; they arouse no fear or apprehension in us and therefore become automatic. Yet they still serve very important purposes in our lives and enable us to remember things, to communicate with others or to organise our lives in a particular way. While the rules for these are not so apparent, we still work within certain conventions, many of which we set up for ourselves. For instance, do you have your own form of shorthand when taking notes? Do you write your shopping list in a certain way? I know that I do, and do so consciously. My shopping list is organised in groups of things that will be stocked together on the shelves of the supermarket – fruit and vegetables in one column, tinned goods in another, a separate list for cleaning products, another group for paper goods and so on. This not only enables me to be more efficient when I'm shopping, but also jogs my memory for other things in the same section or group of products.

So, why do some rules for writing appear so intimidating, while others are simply part of the way we are? Part of the explanation here has to do with familiarity – the more we do, the easier it becomes. Good examples of this are learning to drive a car or ride a bicycle. We get to the stage where we do things without consciously thinking about them: to a certain extent, automatic pilot takes over. This is not, of course, restricted to writing, but affects everything else we do in our lives. It will certainly be so for you starting out in your chosen profession. At first, everything you do is a mystery and appears to be governed by rules that you have yet to take on board and internalise as part of the way you work. These rules need to be learned and, once they are, they make your life easier and less of a mystery.

To a certain extent, the same is true of writing. If you successfully learn the rules of essay writing, for instance, it is more likely that you will have success in what you achieve. In terms of reflective writing, there is tremendous scope for creating your own rules and strategies as well as using those already created by others.

## What kind of writer are you?

We often think that the way that we do things is the way that everyone does them.

Understanding how and why we write enables us to select ways of writing that may help us in reflecting. Sharples suggests that writers can be divided by the two broad approaches that they take to their writing – Discoverers and Planners.

Discoverers, he says, are:

*driven by engagement with the text. For them, self-understanding arises from writing. They may prefer to begin by scribbling out a draft that reveals their thoughts to them. Then, they often rework their text many times, reading and revising until it 'shapes up' to the constraints of the task and audience. The rhythm of their writing is often one of long periods of engaged composing, followed by extensive revision.*

Sharples 1999, p. 112

In contrast, planners:

*are driven by reflection. For these people, writing flows from understanding. They spend a large proportion of their time on exploring ideas and on preparing mental or written plans. The plans guide composing and when there is a mismatch they either edit the text or revise the plan. Their rhythm of composing is, typically, one of rapid alternation between engagement and reflection, continually making minor adjustments to keep plan and text in harmony.*

Sharples 1999

It is, of course, rare that we would all fall neatly into one category or the other. But, you may recognise some of your own characteristics from these descriptions. But how will this help with our own writing? By recognising the ways that we have approached writing in the past, we can anticipate the ways in which we can make writing work for us. Equally, we can weigh up different ways of approaching writing and make a reasoned decision that some of them are not for us. This is really important in being comfortable with your writing, in choosing to write rather than being compelled to write because you are expected to. By understanding your own relationship with writing you are more likely to view it as a positive way of learning rather than something that is imposed upon you by an outside force.

Sharples (1999) goes further in his identification of writing styles by citing a study by Wyllie (1993) who looked at student and academic writers and attempted to classify them by the strategies they used as writers. This is shown in Table 2.5.

Table 2.5 **Classification of writing strategies** (adapted from Sharples 1999, from original work by Wyllie 1993)

| Writing characteristics | Watercolourist | Architect | Bricklayer | Sketcher | Oil painter |
|---|---|---|---|---|---|
| Overall type of writer | Planner | Planner (external) | Planner/discoverer | Discoverer/planner | Discoverer |
| Strategy for writing | Single draft of whole paper with minimal revision, usually sequential | Plan mostly before writing, then write, then review | Polish one sentence, paragraph or section before moving to the next | Rough plan, revise later | Jot down ideas as they occur, organise later, rarely sequential |
| Strategy for planning | Plan in head with broad headings | Detailed plan. Compose with broad headings | Type of planning depends on combination of strategies | Compose with broad headings | Compose with broad headings. Sometimes have a rough plan |
| Order of writing | Always sequential | Often sequential | Sometimes sequential | Sometimes sequential, sometimes jump about | Sometimes sequential, sometimes jump about |
| Starting writing | Rarely start easiest part first | Sometimes start easiest part first | Rarely starts easiest part first | Occasionally start the easiest part first | Often start easiest part first |
| Revision strategy | Little revision - some changes | Revise a fair amount, mainly at sentence level | Fair amount of revision, mainly spelling, grammar and re-sequencing | Much revision, mainly meaning and sequence changes, and sentence level | Much revision, particularly meaning and sentence |
| Correction strategy | Tend not to correct | Rarely correct as they go, mainly on printout | Correct at both stages, but mainly later | Correct as they go, also later | Correct as they go, but mainly later |
| Strategy for reviewing work | Tend to review more on screen than other strategies | Tend to review on printout | Will review on screen, but prefer printout | Review on screen and on printout | Least tendency to review on screen, mainly printout |
| Relationship with screen | Don't find screen restrictive; rarely lose overall sense of the text | Occasionally find screen too restrictive | Often find screen restrictive. Often lose overall sense of the text | Occasionally find screen restrictive | Occasionally find screen restrictive |

## Reflective activity

Think about the ways that you approach your writing. Using Table 2.5, tick the features that most apply to you. The column that contains the most ticks will show your writing tendencies.

This table illustrates what we all really know at heart – that different people approach writing in different ways. But sometimes we need reminding of this. Why do some people appear to sit effortlessly at a word processor, or with pen and paper in front of them, and write thousands of words, when the rest of us make just one more cup of coffee or hang another load of washing on the line, putting off the moment when we have to sit down with an empty screen in front of us! The different strategies identified by Wyllie may help us to understand the creative processes we use in writing. In order to accept that we can all be equally successful in writing we need to find a way of writing that suits us, rather than attempting to conform to one that someone else imposes.

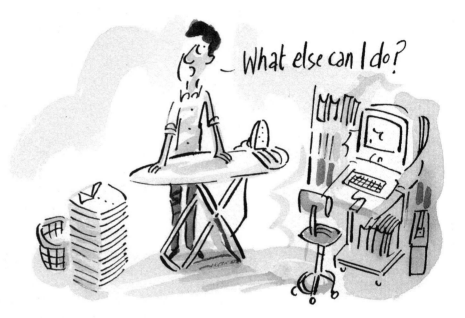

*If you pick the wrong approach for you, it's all too easy to delay writing*

## Reflective activity

Return to the list of types of writing in the first activity. For each one, identify whether you enjoyed this type of writing, whether you disliked it or whether you have no real emotion about it.

Think about the types of writing you have enjoyed in the past. These might be where you have got pleasure or satisfaction from writing or where you have gained from the experience of writing, even although the actual act of doing it may have been difficult for you. What was it about these that made them enjoyable?

Now consider the list of the types of writing that you don't enjoy. What is it about these that you don't like?

Knowing the reasons why you have enjoyed writing are important because you can plan to write reflectively in a style that suits you, and you feel comfortable with. For instance, if you like to write with a definite structure to your writing that has been framed for you, you may like to utilise one or more of the reflective strategies outlined in this book. This brings us back to whether you fall into the category of being a discoverer or a planner. For many people the idea of writing to a pre-determined structure is what puts them off, because they find it difficult to reduce their experiences into categories. For them, the types of writing that depend on creating a self made structure, such as writing a letter, a story or a poem might be more attractive. Similarly, you may find that one single strategy is not appropriate for all of the times that you want to write, and it is useful to consider trying other ways of writing that appear to be better suited to what you are writing about.

### Choosing to write reflectively

Writing can be used as a strategy in itself for reflection. In this case remember that it is the reflective component that is key here – that in writing reflectively you are writing to learn; to enable you to take another perspective. This is hard work; you will be deliberately deciding to explore your own reality and own experiences and at times this may be painful or reveal things to you that have previously been hidden. Equally, there can be great joy in writing, when we unlock secrets that have puzzled us for some time, or that we learn things about ourselves and those around us that we like and can celebrate. You will find strategies for reflective writing in Chapter 5.

## Challenges to writing

We often have a reluctance to write – think back to that list of types of writing that you didn't enjoy and the reasons that you gave for these. There are numerous reasons why we might put up barriers to writing, and unless you write habitually through choice, for instance keeping a diary, the act of writing tends to be something that we do because others tell us to do it. There are many barriers (and often excuses!) that we put up about writing, which we allow to inhibit us in seeing writing as a positive strategy for learning. Some of the reasons for this lie in the features of writing that we perceive to be outside of our control.

### Rules for writing

We talked earlier about the 'rules' of writing. We may have been put off writing as a result of 'rules' being externally imposed – rules such as what you are expected to write about and how you are supposed to write it. This means that the writing tended not to be under our own control, we were writing to a formula that wasn't really very satisfying because it lacked an individual component.

Our experiences of writing are mainly a result of our past educational experiences or our need to write within the confines in our professional role – we learned to write for other people, and we write what others want us to write in the style others expect. In other words we learn-to-write through the processes of socialisation and teaching. These serve important purposes in enabling us to achieve what we need in order to get to the next stage in our lives, such as passing exams or successfully applying for a job, where we need to know the specific rules of writing in that particular setting. We learn the externally imposed rules of writing for other people but don't necessarily develop our own writing style.

You will also have been 'taught' the rules of writing as a formal process for communication – these rules become so ingrained that it is difficult for us to conceive of writing we can understand if it doesn't follow these rules. For instance, think back to the first time you opened a set of case notes. They would have been written in an order, and often language, that was not familiar to you, and thus you probably understood very little of what was written. However, once the conventions being used were explained to you, you would be able to make more sense of them, and eventually adopt the same sort of writing style yourself. So we are taught not only how to write but the ways in which to write it and often even what to write. This is because writing for this purpose becomes a medium of communication, so all people reading the notes and adding to them need to understand the set of rules governing the writing used within them.

Earlier, we asked you to identify as many types of writing as you could that were governed by different rules. Can you now add to these? The rules can be seen in a positive as well as a negative way because, once we understand them, they provide us with the structure and boundaries for what we write in a certain situation. These are useful, because they mean that anyone who knows the rules can understand what is expected and what is written. For instance, once you learn the rules of deciphering essay questions, and how essays are structured, then you will have little difficulty in writing work that gains a pass grade. At other times, however, you may be able to write without rules, such as when you are writing only for yourself and no-one else is likely to see the result. You may also have the freedom of writing where you define the structure, because you are not expected to conform to a given way of writing – this might be in a learning journal or a diary, for instance. Although others may read this, they do not have the power to ask you to write in a particular way.

In writing reflectively, as part of your reflective practice, you will meet all three approaches. In required course work, for instance, you may be asked to use a particular framework for reflection, or the choice may be left to you, with the proviso that you do use a recognised strategy. You may also be required to keep a learning journal, or portfolio, that is structured in a specific way and is used by all the people on your course. This is usually done so that you can concentrate on the reflective activity itself rather than having to find a structure to your writing as well. As you get to the later stages in the course, and you are more familiar with what you are doing in terms of having 'learned the rules' of the reflective process, you may be able to select alternative ways of writing reflectively.

However, you may also be writing reflectively in private. And here there are no rules other than the ones that you impose on yourself. Many students, especially when they are starting out, choose to use a specific strategy or framework. Others, however, may write instinctively as it suits them. This all comes back to the kind of writing style you have. The important criterion is that, no matter what you select in terms of your rules for writing, it should help you to achieve what you need to.

### Writing for others

Allen *et al.* (1989) suggest that we *learn-to-write* primarily for other people, not for ourselves. This can be seen as fundamental to why many of us do not see the value of writing reflectively. Our previous experiences of writing have been rooted in providing some sort of evidence to others that we have learned something. This is opposite to the concept that writing might be useful in helping us to understand the world through a creative process of writing for ourselves. This idea of learning-to-write is based on several assumptions:

- We can learn content whether or not we can write well
- Writing and thinking involve different skills; therefore one is not necessarily linked to the other
- Knowing something logically comes before writing about it
- Writing is a sequential, linear activity that involves mastery of components such as sentence construction or outlining
- Communication is the main purpose of writing; therefore, for students, written work is a product in which the student reports what he or she already knows
- The student's audience is most often assumed to be the teacher.

**Keywords**

**Paradigm**
A collection of features that together provide a particular view on something, e.g. the quantitative and qualitative paradigms in research

These explain a great deal in terms of understanding why writing is, for most of us, not an activity that we use creatively in our learning. Writing is usually an end point, when we finally pull all our reading and thinking together into an essay or other form of writing that will be given to others for their assessment and approval. None of the features in this list involves students writing for themselves; hence, to some extent, writing may be seen as something that is not for us at all and therefore is only done when others demand it of us. In fact, it might not even be viewed as a useful activity, other than as a part of passing course components as a means to an end – a necessary evil to be got through and then not done again unless others require it.

For most of us, our experiences of writing are located within the *learning-to-write* framework. On the whole, we wrote what we thought others wanted us to write – for instance we would rewrite from textbooks in order to show a teacher that we had read (but not necessarily understood or learned) the material; or we would write an exam paper to prove that we could remember what we had read or been told. At times you may have written an essay with a title that asked you to discuss ideas, or analyse, or even be creative – but the title might have been given to you by someone else. Moreover, your success would have been dependent upon you correctly decoding the unseen rules about what was being asked of you – for instance, how many times have you been pleased with an essay, only to have it returned with a disappointing grade and the comment 'You haven't answered the question'. The *learning-to-write* **paradigm** assumes that thinking and writing are separate and different processes and that writing is simply a means to an end, not the end in itself.

---

## *Reflective activity*

### Why do you do what you do?

Think back to your school days. Try to describe your attitude to writing as a child. Why did you write, who did you write for?

What are the messages that your childhood experiences have given you about the value and purpose of writing that you have carried with you into your adult life?

Now think about your educational experiences, and other writing that you have done since school. Did this reinforce those previous experiences of writing, or enable you to develop different skills?

What is your attitude to writing now?

There is, though, another way of looking at writing that enables us to see it as under our control and writing for ourselves. It is this attitude that enables us to use writing as a personal strategy for learning from our experiences, as opposed to the writing that we do for others. This idea of *writing-to-learn* assumes the following things:

- Writing is a process through which content is learned or understood (as opposed to memorised or reported)
- Writing skills are primarily thinking skills (competence in one is inseparable from competence in the other)
- Writing is a process of developing an understanding or coming to know something
- Writing is a dialectical, recursive process rather than a linear or sequential one
- Higher order conceptual skills can only evolve through a writing process in which the writer engages in an active, on-going dialogue with him or herself and others – learning and discovery are purposes as important for writing as communication
- Different disciplines use different conceptual processes and thus have different standards for writing. Students can best learn writing within their own disciplines while writing for real, concrete audiences.

Adapted from Allen *et al.* 1989, p. 7

In contrast to the *learning-to-write* paradigm, this view suggests that the very process of writing is seen as a way of learning. This assumes that writing and thinking happen at the same time; that writing comes from thinking and that creativity arises from thinking about and doing writing. An important point here is that the *writing-to-learn* paradigm links understanding with writing. It suggests that we learn as a result of interacting with the subject matter and that in the process this material becomes transformed into 'knowing'. Thus, the very process of writing is not seen as a passive activity but is dynamic and leads to new connections being made and new understanding occurring.

These features are important when we see reflective writing as part of our strategy for learning about our practice in a professional capacity, because they acknowledge the individual nature of writing for each person. They remove the idea of writing from the basic idea of writing for others, producing a way of combining thinking and writing in a dialogue with ourselves to develop our understanding and create knowledge out of our experience.

We need, therefore, to see writing as being under our own control, and to see that we write for ourselves, not for other people. This is a

## RRRRRRapid recap

Check your progress so far by working through each of the following questions.

1. What is a SWOB analysis?
2. Where do our professional values come from?
3. How can knowing your preferred learning style help you to learn more effectively?
4. What are the challenges to using writing to learn?

If you have difficulty with more than one of the questions, read through the section again to refresh your understanding before moving on.

## References

Allen, D.G., Bowers, B. and Diekelmann, N. (1989) Writing to learn: a reconceptualisation of thinking and writing in the nursing curriculum. *Journal of Nursing Education*, **28**, 6–11.

Kolb, D.A. (1984) *Experiential Learning: Experience as the source of learning and development.* Prentice Hall, Englewood Cliffs, NJ.

Sharples, M. (1999) *How We Write.* London: Routledge.

Wyllie, R. (1993) *On the road to discovery: a study of the composing strategies of academic writers using the word processor.* University of Lancaster, MA thesis.

# Frameworks for reflection

## Learning outcomes

By the end of this chapter you should be able to:

- Recognise a number of frameworks for reflection
- Work through some of your own experiences using these frameworks
- Create 'model' critical incident analyses from your own experience

In this chapter we introduce you to structures and strategies for reflection that you can choose to use in which ever way you want, whether with other people or by yourself. We call all of these by the umbrella term 'frameworks' to avoid confusion. Although this is quite a theoretical chapter, each framework will be illustrated with examples to enable you to see how it works in practice. We will also be analysing the frameworks that we are using, so you can see how they have arisen, the ways in which they can be used and how they compare to each other. We hope that you will see that structures and strategies can be useful as a guide, especially when starting out, because they provide cues, and ways of breaking experiences down that may be new to you. But, all of these frameworks are simply that. It is up to you to put your own stamp on them, to adjust them to suit your purposes so that they can be used effectively in the way you want. Ultimately, there is no one right way of reflecting, in the same way that there is usually more than one way of doing most things. We hope that the frameworks presented in this chapter will provide you with a range of strategies that will help you to look outside your usual ways of thinking and operating. We hope you will see that this can be liberating and broaden perspectives on the ways that we experience life.

Many models and frameworks for reflection have been developed, and of necessity we have chosen to present and explore three of these in detail. These are the ones you will come across most commonly, both in your educational experiences and in your reading. However, we hope that these will whet your appetite to explore further and really expand the strategies that you use to learn from and develop your practice. It may be that for coursework purposes you are restricted in the strategies you use to those provided by your lecturers. However, this does not stop you experimenting, particularly in the work that you do by yourself – in your reflective journal or personal critical reflection work, for instance. Perhaps you could try new strategies working with your mentors and supervisors in practice?

They may be familiar with a larger range of frameworks that they can introduce you to and help you to explore.

## Using Goodman's levels of reflection

We briefly introduced you to Goodman's levels of reflection in Chapter 1. Here we want to develop these further to show you how you will gradually increase the depth and breadth of your reflective work through your course.

### First level reflection

When you begin your reflective practice you will only be expected to be working at Goodman's first level (Goodman 1984). This expects your work to be largely descriptive, where you concentrate on getting down the basic facts of what happened and show some awareness of what was going on at the time. Goodman suggests that at this level you will be reflecting in order to reach given objectives. These can be seen as relating to efficiency, effectiveness and accountability for one's actions.

Sometimes these accounts will read more as a story than as a piece of academic work. However, your assessor/supervisor will only be looking for evidence that you can identify the features of the incident you are describing and that you have learned something from it as a result. An example of this is given in the following case study.

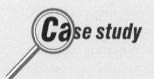

**Case study**

### First level reflection

I arrived on the ward at 7.30 ready to begin a 12-hour shift. After receiving handover, my mentor assigned me the job of bathing Mr B with the help of a health-care assistant. Mr B has Creutzfeldt–Jakob disease (CJD), a progressive disease of the nervous system with rapid deterioration due to spongiform encephalopathy. He is not expected to live until Christmas, even though he is only 19 years old. He is mentally aware of what is going on but is physically unable to demonstrate activities of daily living, including eating and drinking, has limited communication skills and is doubly incontinent. He is unsafe on his feet so mobilises with a wheelchair.

I approached Mr B's bed and asked his consent to take him for a bath. While the bath was running we began helping him to undress. He looked rather nervous – I think it was because he was having two young female nurses caring for his personal needs. As he usually has his mother looking after him, he must have felt a little uncomfortable. At the thought of myself being in his position, being the same age as him, I began to feel embarrassed too.

I thought that I could not possibly be a professional individual if I let my embarrassment and sympathy get in the way of my nursing care.

We assisted Mr B into the bath and started his wash. I knew he was uncomfortable and wanted to be able to wash himself, but was unable to do so. I was finding it difficult to look him in the eye, especially when it came to washing his genitalia, because at this stage he was getting increasingly embarrassed. I tried to ease this by making conversation, but in a way this made things worse because I felt I was being patronising in what I was saying. Although physically he is helpless his mind is still fully active.

After the bath we dried Mr B, dressed him and returned him in the wheelchair to bed. To the health care assistant it was another job done, but the feelings I had afterwards, as I am sure was the case with Mr B, stayed with me for some time.

This example presents a good descriptive account of both what happened and the nurse's part in this. She incorporates her feelings about what was happening at the time, but does not go much beyond this, other than in equating her feelings with the patient's and thinking a little about the role of a nurse. In this way she achieves her objectives in exploring her reaction to the experience. She identifies her efficiency, in that the task was achieved. She questions whether she was really effective as a nurse because, although the bath itself was completed, she felt she had not addressed Mr B's psychological and emotional needs. She recognises her accountability as a student nurse and sees this as being more than that expected from a support worker.

Reflective accounts at this level may be used as the basis for discussion with your supervisor, or perhaps in a classroom situation with your colleagues. You may also start to build a bank of these in a portfolio as evidence of your beginning work as a reflective practitioner. But, as you get further on in your course, you will be expected to become more analytical in this kind of work and start to present conclusions. This is where you will move to Goodman's second level.

## Second level reflection

At this level, you will be starting to identify your learning and drawing conclusions about patient care that are transferable to other situations. You will be using theoretical concepts to explore and explain what has happened, and to provide you with further insight and understanding. In short, you will be creating your own knowledge base by applying theory to practice, and considering theory in the light of practice. Goodman suggests that reflection at this level shows awareness of the implications of both personal and professional values in addition to identifying the rationale and evidence basis of actions taken. An example of reflection at this level is shown in the case study below.

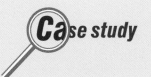

## Second level reflection

Mrs James had been admitted to the ward following a fall and had multiple bruising and cuts to her body. Throughout her time on the ward she had been mildly confused, with a tendency to wander unsupervised. As stated by McConnell (1998), this is a major concern for nurses within hospitals and care facilities. We were told that Mrs James was unsteady on her feet and should not attempt to walk on her own without assistance. This is reinforced by the work of Oliver *et al.* (cited by Kinn and Hood 2001) who say that greater disability may result from anxiety and loss of confidence following a fall.

On the day of the event we had noticed that Mrs James was particularly agitated. This could have been a behavioural cue that she was in pain (Husband 2002). We asked her the problem, and administered analgesics when she confirmed our suspicions. She settled back onto her bed. Shortly after this she rang the call bell and told me of her continuing discomfort, wanting further pain relief. I explained that the tablets she had been given would take some time to take effect and that she should stay on her bed as they might make her drowsy. As Desbien and Wu (2000, cited by Husband 2002) suggest, I was aware that elderly patients often pay little regard to the side effects associated with pain relief.

I began to walk away, but was called back by Mrs James. I felt slightly annoyed, because of the time I had taken in explaining the situation to her. However, as I turned to respond, Mrs James fell to the floor, hitting her face heavily.

Initially I froze with the shock of seeing her falling, and then I felt panic about what I should be doing. This was the first time I had witnessed a patient falling and because of my lack of medical knowledge and inexperience I was scared by it and did not know what to do. I called for help.

My inclination was to help Mrs James to her feet, but the staff nurse said to leave her where she was as she might have further injuries. This can include hip fractures, 25% of which occur in the elderly in acute care settings (Stone 1994). I have found since that over 30% of patients aged 65 and over experience at least one serious fall each year (Sowden and Dickson 1996, cited by Kinn and Hood 2001). 84% of these accidents occur in an acute care setting (McConnell 1998).

This incident has helped me to draw understanding from the situation. While I felt guilty initially because I felt the incident was my fault, I have realised that health authorities see falls as an 'unavoidable problem' (Sweeting 1994, cited by Kinn and Hood 2001), highlighting to me that within my situation there may be very little that could have been done in the way of prevention.

Reflecting on this incident has enabled me to develop my understanding of ways of minimising falls in the elderly, and prepared me to respond effectively and correctly if they do. My primary objective is to be armed with the knowledge of what to do so that I can respond more quickly. I need to be more effective at communicating with confused patients. I also need to understand more about risk assessment, which aims to establish the levels of care required, along with areas of caution, and can be seen as fundamental to all patient care (Royal College of Nursing, cited by Parboteeah 2002).

*Case study continued*

### References

Husband, L. (2002) Caring for the patient in pain, in *Common Foundation Studies in Nursing*, 3rd edn (eds N. Kenworthy, G. Snowley and C. Gilling). Churchill Livingstone, Edinburgh, pp. 457–480.

Kinn, S. and Hood, K. (2001) A falls risk-assessment tool in an elderly care environment. *British Journal of Nursing*, **10**, 440–449.

McConnell, E.A. (1998) Managing patient falls and wandering. *Nursing Management*, **9**, 75.

Parboteeah, S. (2002) Safety in practice, in *Foundations of Nursing Practice: Making the difference*, 2nd edn (eds R. Hogston and M.P. Simpson). Palgrave Macmillan, Basingstoke, pp. 55–102.

Stone, M. (1994) Falls and fractures: an institutional problem. *Geriatric Medicine*, **10**, 15–17.

This student shows how his experience has triggered a need to go and develop his understanding through reading. In turn this is reflected back into practice as he develops his action plan for what he can do should he meet the situation again. He is moving confidently between theory and practice here so that his actions are underpinned by his knowledge. He also demonstrates the beginnings of his awareness of his role as a professional practitioner, bound by personal and professional beliefs of what role a nurse should take. He was concerned that this accident occurred while the patient was under his care, and, identifying a knowledge deficit, wanted to ensure that he had the understanding to prevent harm occurring in future. He is clearly demonstrating the ability to transfer his learning from this one case out to general principles for dealing with similar situations.

## Third level reflection

Finally, Goodman's third level includes an acknowledgement of the wider influences of ethical and political influences on care delivery. This takes the reflective activity one stage further by relating the parameters of care to societal norms and constraints, such as health policy, health economics and resources. The following case study illustrates how a lack of resources can inhibit optimum care.

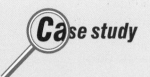

### Case study

### Third level reflection

Having assessed Mr Sheppard's mobility at home I returned to the office to place the order for grab rails to be put in the bathroom and for a stair lift to get him upstairs. There was no possibility of moving the bed downstairs because of the room available.

I am so frustrated!

Here is a man blocking a much needed elderly care bed who cannot go home because of a lack of resources to supply and fit simple mobility aids. We have the grab rails, but fitting will be delayed for a month because of a lack of carpenters at Social Services. The chair lift is out of the question until after April (6 months away) because the budget for such things has already been spent. The couple are unable to afford a lift themselves and they are reluctant to go to charities for help.

### A week later

Having followed this incident further I have come to an understanding of the situation. We do not live in a society where everything is free and available on demand, although this is often the impression that we get. Social Services have a budget allocated to home aids and resourcing their fitting. There is no more money available for this once the budget has been allocated. They have only two carpenters and one is on long-term sick leave, so the waiting list for fitting grab rails is necessarily long. So, what are the alternatives? I talked to Mr and Mrs Sheppard about re-arranging downstairs so that a single bed can be brought into the living room, and they have got their son-in-law to do this. The room has been made safe by removing slip rugs and clutter from the floor, and trailing leads. The lighting has been improved with spotlights and higher-voltage bulbs. As Mrs Sheppard is the principal carer, and physically sound, we have decided to ask the Red Cross to provide a commode that she can empty in the bathroom upstairs. I have talked with the GP about care help for washing and bathing so that Mrs Sheppard can have a break. Mr Sheppard will be going home in a couple of days – 3 weeks earlier than would have been possible if we had waited for the rails to be fitted.

This is not an ideal solution, but is the best possible given the circumstances.

This excerpt omits the theoretical exploration and justification that was present in the original in order to illustrate the third-level criteria of considering the political and social context of care. This Occupational Therapy student had assumed that resources are unlimited and were available dependent on need. This was an extremely valuable lesson for her, as she not only found alternatives to the problem that were workable and practical, she also realised

### Reflective activity

Think about the reflective work that you have already done – whether as part of your course, as a result of completing activities from this book or in other parts of your life. Which levels of reflection have you been working at? What would you need to do to move to the next level(s)?

early in her career that care is not value-free but is dependent upon societal values and priorities, which may not be in the interests of every individual.

All these levels can be used within any of the strategies and frameworks for reflection that you will use. We now present three frameworks, illustrated with case studies, to help you to explore and understand how structures can help you in starting off your reflective practice.

## Gibbs's reflective cycle

The first framework we explore has been developed from Kolb's ideas in educational theory and develops the features of the ERA cycle. This is the reflective cycle developed by Graham Gibbs (1988) and is shown in Figure 3.1.

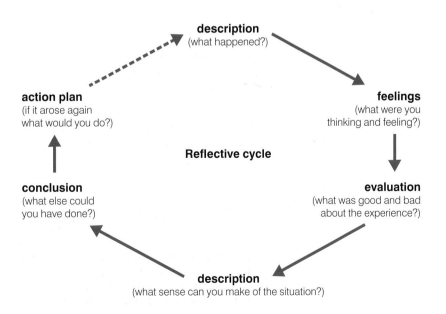

**Figure 3.1** *Gibbs's reflective cycle (1988)*

○━┓ *Keywords*

**Seminal**
Important, influencing
later developments

Gibbs's framework has achieved the status of a **seminal** theory in reflective practice and it would be difficult to find any paper or textbook on reflective practice written in the past 15 years that did not draw on his work in some way. Gibbs's cycle consists of six stages that guide you through the stages of the reflective process by asking a series of cue questions. Prior to this, the critical incident to be reflected on must have been chosen (see Chapter 1).

## Stage 1: Description of the event

The starting point is to write down, or tell someone else, a potted version of the event that you want to reflect on. The type of event that you select will depend on whether you want to share this with someone else or whether, at this time, you need to keep it to yourself. At this stage, it is important to get as much down about the event as you possibly can, and in as objective a way as you can. Some of the things that you might want to include are:

- Where were you?
- Who else was there?
- Why were you there?
- What were you doing?
- What were the other people doing?
- What was the context of the event?
- What happened?
- What was your part in this?
- What parts did the other people play?
- What was the result?

## Stage 2: Feelings

At this stage you try to recall, and explore, the things that were going on inside your head. These are often the things that cause us to feel happy, or dissatisfied with the event, and why it sticks in our mind in the first place. This is also the stage which you might find difficult to share with other people. Some questions that are useful here are:

- How were you feeling when the event started?
- What were you thinking at the time?
- What were you thinking about when it happened?
- How did it make you feel then?
- What did other people's actions/words make you think?

**Keywords**

**Evaluation**
Assessing the worth or value of something, to measure it against a standard

- What did these make you feel?
- How did you feel about the outcome of the event?
- What do you think about it now?
- List the emotions that you have gone through from the start to the finish of the event
- Which of these is most significant or important to you?

## Stage 3: Evaluation

When we evaluate something we give it a value, or measure it against some sort of a standard. What we are trying to do is to arrive at some sort of judgement about what has happened so that we can recognise all of its components, and not just those that are at the front of our minds when we think of it. So, the sorts of question that we might ask here are:

- What was good about the experience?
- What was bad about the experience, or didn't go so well?

## Stage 4: Analysis

This means 'to break things down into their component parts' so that they can be explored separately. So we need to ask more detailed questions about the answers to the last stage. We might ask such questions as:

- What went well?
- What did I do well?
- What did others do well?
- What went wrong, or did not turn out the way I thought it should?
- In what ways did I contribute to this?
- In what ways did others contribute to this?
- Why might these things have happened?

## Stage 5: Conclusion

This differs from the evaluation stage in that now you have explored the issue from different angles and have a great deal more information on which to base your judgement. It is here that you are likely to develop insight into your own and other people's behaviour in terms of how they contributed to the outcome of the event. Sometimes this is difficult, because we may realise that the way we handled an event, or our part in it, might not have been the most effective way of going about things. This, however, is exactly the point! Remember, the purpose of reflection is to learn from experience. Without the detailed analysis and honest exploration that occurs during these stages, it is unlikely that all aspects of the event will be taken into account, and therefore valuable opportunities for learning can be missed. Gibbs suggests that we ask ourselves what we could have done differently as part of this stage.

### Stage 6: Action plan

At this stage you are invited to think yourself forward into encountering the event again, and to plan what you would do – would you act differently, or would you be likely to do the same again?

Gibbs' cycle stops here, with anticipated action. The cycle is completed tentatively by suggesting that the next time the event occurs it will be the focus of another reflective cycle. This whole cycle is illustrated in the case study below.

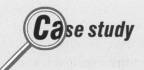
**Case study**

### Sarah – a student physiotherapist

**Description – what happened?**

I had been asked by my supervisor to work with Mrs Simpson, an 83-year-old lady in for respite care to give her daughter a break from the day-to-day caring routine. Despite her senile dementia, it was hoped that we would be able to increase her mobility and self-care activities so that she wasn't just a physical drain on her daughter. I was hoping to do some passive stretching exercises with her, before getting her walking with her frame. My supervisor, Jackie, was working with other patients on the ward, doing pre-op breathing exercises.

Mrs Simpson was with three other patients grouped together at the far end of a Nightingale-type ward and separated from the other patients, who were predominantly in for day surgery. I had worked with all four patients before and had no worries as I approached Mrs Simpson, although I had been on the receiving end of her extensive foul and abusive language before. Mrs Simpson presented all members of the caring team with challenges every day, as even the most simple of tasks, such as getting out of bed and taking medicines, were met with refusal, swearing and insulting behaviour.

That morning, Mrs Simpson was dressed and sitting on a chair beside her bed. I drew the curtains around the bedspace, and positioned everything ready to help her back on to the bed so that we could do some exercises. I was talking to her all the time, but got no verbal response at all. As I bent down to support her in standing up, I felt a sudden sharp scrape down the side of my face. Mrs Simpson began to swear quite loudly at me and I was worried that the other patients and staff would hear the shouting and wonder what was going on. I tried to reassure her, but she scratched me again, pulling her nails down the side of my cheek. I was really shocked and, never having been physically attacked before, my first thoughts were to get someone else to help. I ensured Mrs Simpson was safely in her chair, drew back the curtains and went to find help.

*Case study continued*

### Feelings – what were you thinking and feeling?

Initially, my feelings at the time were for Mrs Simpson, as I was concerned that my actions had caused her to feel threatened and strike out to defend herself. I felt guilty, but stayed calm and tried to think what I had done wrong. I felt embarrassed but Jackie was very supportive and reassured me that it wasn't my fault. A few minutes later though I felt very cold and started shaking. I found it difficult that someone I was trying to help would attack me.

### Evaluation – what was good and bad about the experience?

I had prepared for the therapy session with Mrs Simpson by reviewing her physio records, and reading the nursing notes when I got to the ward. I had also talked to the Staff Nurse looking after her that morning to find out how she was and whether there had been anything happening that might affect my work with her. Nothing indicated that Mrs Simpson was in an aggressive mood that morning. I had also planned what I was going to do in advance. I made sure that I introduced myself, and talked all the time to Mrs Simpson, telling her in advance about what I was doing and what the plans were. I drew the curtains to ensure privacy for the transfer to the bed and the exercises.

What was bad was that I was sworn at and ended up getting scratched on my face. As a result I had to go to Occupational Health and have the wound cleaned properly and a tetanus update, then I went home as I was still shocked, so I missed the rest of my clinical experience that day, which I was looking forward to.

I was working by myself at the end of the ward, in a section divided off by a solid division, and thus was out of immediate hearing of the other staff. I also attempted to transfer Mrs Simpson by myself.

### Analysis – what sense can you make of the situation?

The result was that we decided not to proceed with the physio that day, so I felt guilty and upset that my actions resulted in the patient not being treated. I felt a failure, that I wasn't able to do the job I was expected to do, and as a result the patient suffered. However, Mrs Simpson had no recollection of what she had done to me, because of her dementia, and perhaps this was a good thing as it meant that I could go back into her room the next day to continue her therapy. I realised that Mrs Simpson hadn't deliberately meant to hurt me, but that this kind of aggressive behaviour is a result of the dementia and was a way of her protecting herself when she felt threatened. Since the incident I have read more about confusion, aggression and dementia, and realise that it always has to be anticipated in patients of this kind, especially when they are not in their familiar environment. I have also suggested to the University that we have some sessions included early in our training about defusing a potentially violent situation, self-defence and breakaway techniques. It would be useful to explore the psychology of being attacked and ways in which we can deal with it and come to terms with it.

I realised that my reactions later, after I had made sure she was safe, were symptoms of shock. I felt very vulnerable and at risk myself, but understand now, after talking it through with Jackie, that this is a normal reaction designed to enable us to cope with stressful situations.

### Conclusion – what else could you have done?

I realise now that there wasn't a lot that I could have done in that situation anyway, and perhaps the best thing was to leave Mrs Simpson to calm down. I did wonder whether I could have done something else in that position and what other choices I had in trying to do what I was supposed to do. I could have stayed with Mrs Simpson

*Case study continued*

and tried to calm her down, but I didn't have the knowledge or experience for dealing with aggressive patients, and didn't know what to do.

I wonder though, whether it is really a good idea to work with anyone who has a history of aggressive behaviour by yourself. I also feel that I should have spent longer sitting and talking with her before trying to move her, to get her used to me and create a calm atmosphere. She hadn't said a word to me before I tried to move her, and maybe I ought to have taken a cue from this that she wasn't feeling very co-operative.

**Action plan – what would you do if this situation arose again?**

I am now more prepared for patients to be violent. I had always thought before that it wouldn't happen to me, and that the person who was attacked was to blame in some way. I don't think that now. In future, where I know that patients have an aggressive history, or even with demented patients, I will be more on my guard. I will take the time to reassure and talk to the patient and ensure that I get their cooperation. I will also try to avoid working alone in an area or where there are patients who can be aggressive.

**Reflections on writing the critical incident**

While writing this assignment I have been able to re-examine my critical incident properly with adequate time to reflect on every detail of what happened. I have had the opportunity to learn from my mistakes and this will enable me to improve my future patient care and think more about my own safety. Although I concluded that this incident was a negative one, now, on reflection, I see that it was very valuable, especially happening when it did in my course, as I am much more aware of the potential for aggression and violence from patients. This is because I have learned not only about violent patients but also how to use the technique of reflection to help me get through, and understand, what happens in clinical situations. Gibbs's reflective cycle suited this situation because it helped me to break it down and really think about it in a different way. While I hope that I never get attacked again, I do feel that I am more aware of the potential for aggression and have learned to approach situations in a different way from the more naïve attitude that I had before this happened. I have also been prompted to read more about aggression in the NHS, and learn strategies to deal with it. I wouldn't have done this if it hadn't happened to me personally.

Sarah's use of Gibbs's cycle had clearly enabled her both to see the situation in a different way and enabled her to learn for the future. This was obviously a very distressing incident for Sarah, in which she questioned her own actions with a patient and had to face up to her own vulnerability in a situation where she was trying to help. Although the experience itself was negative, the use of Gibbs's cycle enabled her to see the incident in a different way and turn it into a learning experience.

tɔɘɿʈɘЯ*Reflective activity*

The only way to really understand this reflective cycle is to use it yourself to explore something that has happened to you recently. We suggest that you use the questions given at each stage to work your way through an event that has stuck in your mind for some reason. You could choose something arising during your course, or your practical placement, or even something like returning faulty goods to a store or having a conversation with a friend about a problem they have. It is useful to write your reflections down at this stage, especially if you are using an event at work as the focus, as you may be able to use it as part of your portfolio or for some other purpose in your course.

Once you have done that, take a few minutes to think about how you felt doing the exercise.

- How useful did you find Gibbs's cycle?
- How easy was it to use?
- Did you have any difficulties using it?
- Did it enable you to see the event from a wider perspective?
- Did it enable you to reach alternative conclusions about the event to the ones you had when you started out?
- How comfortable did you feeling using it?
- Would you choose to use it again?

Try to give the reasons for your answers to these questions.

Gibbs's approach is characteristic of all the strategies, or frameworks, for reflection that have been developed over the succeeding years. Where Gibbs's reflective cycle stops, however, is at the action planning stage, and this is why we have used a broken line to link it back up to the descriptive stage. What Gibbs has created is a very good framework for the reflective process, i.e. learning from reflecting on something. But it stops at the stage of proposing action. Hence, the reflection can stop, quite legitimately from this point of view, at predicting action in terms of 'If I encountered the situation again, what would I do differently?' Of course, as anyone with even minimal practice experience knows, it is extremely unlikely that another situation will occur that is exactly the same as an experience that you have already had. Experiences may be similar, but they will not be the same. So, although Gibbs provides us with a useful framework for reflecting in the abstract, and usually away from the scene of practice, he does not provide us with the means to close the cycle, nor to move to reflective practice in terms of taking action.

Part of the reason for this lies in the fact that Gibbs's framework arose from an education context, as opposed to a practice basis.

- Gibbs's reflective cycle provides us with a staged framework for working through the exploration of an experience
- It arose as a generalised educational framework and is therefore not focused on practice
- It stops at the stage of framing action

To move from a framework of theoretical reflection to one that arises from a practice environment, and hence is likely to be more useful in clinical contexts, we will move on to the work of Chris Johns.

## Johns's model of structured reflection

Chris Johns's model arose from his work in the Burford Nursing Development unit in the early 1990s. Although it has gone through many developments and presentations since, the 1994 version (presented in Palmer *et al.* 1994) is used here because it is one that is easy to use when beginning reflective practice. Johns himself envisaged this model as being used within a process of guided reflection that has three components:

- Using the model of structured reflection
- Supervision
- Diary structure

Johns says that the model:

*consists of a series of questions which aim to tune the practitioner into her experience in a structured and meaningful way. It emerged as a natural sequence through which practitioners explored their experiences in supervision.*

Johns 1994, cited in Palmer *et al.* 1994, p.112

The framework is presented in Figure 3.2.

The focus for Johns, in developing this framework, was about uncovering and making explicit the knowledge that we use in our practice. So, the framework takes this as its core question, which is explored through the five cue questions. These are further divided into more focused questions to promote detailed reflection. The first two stages of this framework are similar to those we have already considered.

**Core question – What information do I need to access in order to learn through this experience?**

**Cue questions**

**1. Description of the experience**

- Phenomenon – describe the here and now experience
- Causal – what essential factors contributed to this experience?
- Context – what are the significant background factors to this experience?
- Clarifying – what are the key processes (for reflection) in this experience?

**2. Reflection**

- What was I trying to achieve?
- Why did I intervene as I did?
- What were the consequences of my actions for:
    - Myself?
    - The patient/family?
    - The people I work with?
- How did I feel about this experience when it was happening?
- How did the patient feel about it?
- How do I know how the patient felt about it?

**3. Influencing factors**

- What internal factors influenced my decision-making?
- What external factors influenced my decision-making?
- What sources of knowledge did/should have influenced my decision-making?

**4. Could I have dealt with the situation better?**

- What other choices did I have?
- What would be the consequences of these choices?

**5. Learning**

- How do I feel now about this experience?
- How have I made sense of this experience in light of past experiences and future practice?
- How has this experience changed my ways of knowing
    - Empirics
    - Aesthetics
    - Ethics
    - Personal

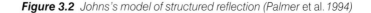

**Figure 3.2** *Johns's model of structured reflection (Palmer et al. 1994)*

## Cue question 1: Description of the experience

At the descriptive stage, Johns provides four cue questions to help structure the description of what has happened. These identify:

- The 'phenomenon' or the experience itself
- The cause of the experience
- The context within which it happened, or the background to it
- 'Clarifying' – at this stage the person is asked to 'put the experience back together and look at it as a whole, identifying the key processes occurring within the experience' (Johns 1994, cited in Palmer *et al.* 1994, p. 113).

As with other frameworks, this sets the scene and provides the baseline for the rest of the reflection. Where it is being used within a supervisory relationship, or for reflecting with other people, it provides an outline of the experience that the other person can understand and work from.

Johns later dropped the four subquestions that structure the description of the experience, because he felt they 'interfered with practitioners telling their stories' (Johns 1998). However, these can be useful for students and practitioners beginning reflection because they help to provide a structure for describing the experience that you might find difficult to do without. Once you become familiar and comfortable with the ways in which you describe your own experiences you may decide that these are no longer necessary.

## Cue question 2: Reflection

At this stage Johns's framework enters the analytical stages, asking the familiar questions about what the person did and felt and what the consequences of the actions and feelings were, and attempts to get them to take the role of the other person in predicting/anticipating their responses.

A difference between Gibbs's and Johns's frameworks here is the question that Johns asks in trying to identify what the person was trying to achieve within the event/incident. This is very important, because it relates to that idea of practicality and context that is missing from Gibbs's framework. We rarely enter a clinical situation without first considering what our intentions are and what we want the results to be. Having already decided on these, we tend to plan our actions to achieve these. Even when we are reflecting on 'on-the-spot' decisions and reactions to things that happen to us, we still fast-track forward in our heads to try to achieve some aim that we can predict. As a result of this, we have something to measure our success (or failure) against, and it is this that creates our sense of satisfaction or dissatisfaction.

> ### Over to you
>
> Look back at Sarah's story in the previous case study. As a practitioner, she certainly had specific aims in mind when she entered her encounter with Mrs Simpson. Can you identify what these might have been? What was it that caused Sarah to be so unhappy with what had happened?

In asking this question, 'What were you trying to achieve within the event/incident?', Johns enables us to identify where the outcomes of an experience do not match up with our intentions. In a clinical situation this is clearly very important, as it enables us to evaluate our performance as practitioners and recognise where we are not achieving what we want to achieve.

Johns also introduces the roles that others have played in the experience at this stage in a more detailed way. Gibbs tends to focus solely on the individual reflecting. For the purposes of this book, 'other people' have been introduced into the cue questions in Gibbs's framework to help you understand further. They are not included in Gibbs's original framework. Johns, however, sees the roles and feelings of others as key to understanding the experience in context. He asks us to think about how the patient was feeling. This can be expanded into identifying how all the other people involved may have been feeling. For instance, there may have been family members, friends or carers with the patient, or other health-care professionals or colleagues involved in the incident. It is important for us to try to take the feelings of others into account when exploring how situations occurred, as we can develop a great deal of insight by considering alternative ways of seeing and experiencing things.

However, there is one word of caution here. Johns does go on to ask us how we know what those other people were feeling. This is a reminder that our perceptions of things may not reflect what the other people were actually feeling. So it is probably useful to explore why we think people were feeling the way we think they were, and checking this out. Many things happen as a result of mistaken perceptions and misunderstandings, so we need to work on recognising where we are making assumptions and where we have evidence to support our conclusions.

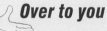

> ## Over to you
>
> What assumptions was Sarah making about how Mrs Simpson was feeling during the incident as a result of it? What was she basing these on?
> Do you think she was right?
> What other explanations can you think of?
> This point, of course, applies to anyone who is involved in an incident that you are reflecting on.

---

> ## Reflective activity
>
> Can you think of an example of your own where you made assumptions about what someone else was thinking and then later found you were wrong?
>
> ● What was the situation?
> ● What assumptions were you making?
> ● Why did you make these?
> ● Did you check them out with the other person?
> ● What did you do on the basis of these assumptions?
> ● What were the consequences?
> ● Were these as you expected – if not why not?
> ● What did you learn as a result of this?

### Cue question 3: Influencing factors

Johns specifically asks you to identify the factors that influenced you within the incident. This cue question uses the analytical and interpretive reflective processes. Here you will be trawling back through your previous knowledge, skills and experience to identify the basis on which you made your decisions and the external factors that may also have had some effect on you.

Internal factors are those that arise from yourself – your previous experiences, any similar cases or situations that you have encountered, intuition, etc.

External factors include any knowledge or information that comes from outside of you – the more objective sources, for instance, such as your reading, guidance from your professional bodies, government policy or your employer's procedures and policies.

This is a useful division for the beginning reflector, because it helps us to separate out what it is we know for ourselves as opposed to what comes from outside of us. It is worth remembering, though, that it

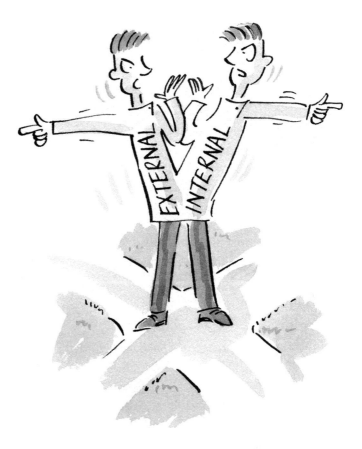

*Each of us is influenced by internal and external factors*

could be said that anything that we know is actually part of us because we have taken it in and perceived it in a way that is unique to us. Although the source of the knowledge may be external, therefore, our use and transformation of it is in many ways unique. The purpose of reflection here then, is to 'unpack' these influences in order to understand, and perhaps challenge, our way of perceiving the world through identifying and acknowledging just what these influences are.

### Cue question 4: Could I have dealt better with the situation?

This stage involves the reflective process of exploring alternatives. Johns's phrasing here assumes that the critical incident being explored was one that could have had a better outcome – it may even have been negative in some way. In later versions of the framework this has changed, as he comes to focus more on how we know what we know, rather than on reflection as a way of changing what we do. Hence, it may be more positive to revert to our phrasing of 'exploring alternatives' here, as a way of widening our perceptions of how we can deal with situations rather than resting with self-criticism and self-improvement.

## Cue question 5: Learning

Finally, Johns asks us, on the basis of the insights gained during the previous stages, to identify what we have learned. He asks us how we now feel about the experience.

Melissa's story presents an incident critical for her, that arose on her first day in placement as a student nurse. It presents a good example of the use of Johns's framework to this stage of the last cue question. Read this now, and then take some time to answer the questions that follow it.

*Case study*

### Melissa – a student nurse

#### Describing the phenomenon

My first placement was on a ward specialising in the surgical care of cardiac patients. Mr Brown, a 68-year-old man, had previously undergone a triple coronary bypass. During the process various drains and catheters, including a central line and chest drain, had been inserted to assist drug administration to and fluid removal from the thoracic cavity. It had been 3 days since Mr Brown's operation; his central line had already been removed but his chest drain was still to be taken out. As a student new to the ward, I was not allowed to do this myself but I was to observe the two staff nurses carry out the procedure.

Mr Brown had been tachycardic (raised heart rate) since his operation, setting off the alarm on the cardiac monitor. Although his raised heart rate was not of concern to the staff, and this had been communicated to Mr Brown, the constant noise coming from the monitor was making Mr Brown very anxious. He started to have anxiety attacks, began to cry and get in an agitated state, increasing his heart and respiration rates even more.

The chest drain was about to be removed but Mr Brown's emotional state created a problem because of his fast breathing and inability to concentrate on what was being said to him. The nurses needed Mr Brown's co-operation in the removal of the drain, but he was too frightened.

As I was not taking part in the procedure, I took it upon myself to calm him down. I sat beside him and held his hand, encouraging him to talk to me in order to take his mind off what was going to happen to him. I told him that removing the drain was the last procedure he would have to undergo and that, although he felt worried, once it was removed he would feel much more comfortable. I also told him that I would be with him through the whole procedure and that it would be over very quickly. I could see that I was having a positive effect on him as his breathing slowed down and he ceased crying. I continued to talk to him and reassured him that the two qualified nurses and I would take care of him. Mr Brown soon slipped into a calm enough state to concentrate on his breathing, the chest drain was then swiftly out and a dressing was applied to the wound.

*Case study continued*

Having not been on a ward before, this was my first major interaction with a patient, and the two nurses involved told me I handled the situation well and contributed to the removal of the drain by helping Mr Brown relax, resulting in his respiration rate slowing down.

### Reflection

When seeing the distress experienced by Mr Brown before the procedure I felt unsettled and worried and instinctively felt that I wanted to help him. I realised I was the person to calm him down – although the nurses calmed him slightly themselves, they were concentrating on the procedure so their attention was not fully centred on Mr Brown's emotional state. Therefore, as I wasn't actively taking part in the removal of the drain, I could give all my attention to him.

I thought my actions were justified: the patient needed to be reassured swiftly or the chest drain could not have been removed as quickly and efficiently and his anxiety would have been prolonged.

During the situation I was faced with many thoughts. Initially I wasn't sure if I was helping. I felt as though I was a hindrance and that my observing the patient might have been making him feel more uncomfortable. When he grasped my hand, though, I realised he was happy for me to be there and was looking to me for reassurance. I felt relieved that I was actually helping and contributing to his care, despite my inexperience and lack of knowledge. He seemed gratified to have me beside him, he felt he wasn't alone and looked upon me as a friend as well as part of the nursing team looking after him. After the drain was removed he said that having a familiar and friendly face certainly made a difference, it made him feel confident and as though he was being taken care of. He said that this, for him, was an important part of nursing.

### Influencing factors

Many internal and external factors influenced my actions. Seeing people distressed unsettles me. I felt uncomfortable with the idea that Mr Brown was suffering from discomfort and wanted to do something to relieve his anxiety. Not being able to help with the procedure, I felt incompetent and helpless just 'observing'. I wanted to take part in one way or another, and having limited nursing skills I realised this was how I could make my contribution.

With Mr Brown feeling distressed, his heart rate was getting higher and higher, and he was aware of this as he could hear it on the monitor. As I didn't know how to interpret the readings on the monitor correctly, the apparent increase on the monitor was making me anxious too, as I thought something serious might happen. My knowledge of cardiac conditions and treatment was very limited so I panicked and thought the situation was worse than it actually was. This was the reason that I reacted in the way that I did. I had previously read that the therapeutic use of touch helps in many ways, and that it can help to build a rapport between nurse and patient, thus bringing about trust in the relationship. By holding his hand I thought reassurance would be provided to let him know that he was not alone, therefore helping to calm him down. Personal experience also made me think that interaction such as kind words and attention between individuals can help relieve a stressful situation.

### Alternative actions

After the nurses and I had finished working with Mr Brown, I didn't think too much about what had happened and wasn't convinced that I had played any role in caring for him. As far as I was concerned, I didn't actually 'do' anything beneficial for the situation. I thought this until one of the staff nurses involved in the procedure, who

*Case study continued*

happened to be my mentor, highlighted to me that I had performed some nursing care with a positive outcome for the patient. Although I didn't physically take part, I successfully supported the patient emotionally through what for him was an emotionally distressing experience.

### Learning

I look back now and realise that I underestimated the use of 'basic' nursing care and that patients' feelings and emotions are equally as important as the reason for their hospitalisation. I now believe that in order for me to become a good nurse in future practice, and to provide holistic care, basic nursing skills have to be learned, before concentrating on the more 'in depth' side of nursing such as medical procedures, treatment and diagnosis.

Having not worked in a nursing environment before, I have no experience to compare this incident to; however, I feel that I have learned a great deal from working with Mr Brown and the nurses involved. Although in this case my feelings of panic were not detected, I have learned that many patients in the future will consider me to be the professional and will expect me to be in control in any situation. A nurse showing panic may unsettle a patient, resulting in lack of confidence and trust. This, in turn, is likely to affect the treatment being given.

As a student with limited experience, I realise that as my course progresses I will become more confident in dealing with situations of this nature. However, increasing my knowledge of some common medical procedures will assist me in future clinical practice as it helps me to understand some of the problems that I may be faced with when implementing treatments.

### Reflections on the use of the framework

By using Johns's reflective model as a guide, I have been able to reflect on the incident and this has enabled me to evaluate the actions that I took during the incident, questioning whether my response was appropriate. It has also allowed me to think of other ways I could have dealt with the situation and the possible outcomes. The reflective strategy has helped me to learn from this experience and has given me an insight into how I might improve my own future practice. It has also shown me that, by continuing the reflective process by following reflective frameworks such as Johns's in future incidents, I may improve the ways of dealing with situations, and acknowledge that I am actually learning something from every experience that I have. The importance of reflection has been reinforced to me in writing up this critical incident, because I hadn't really thought about the importance of emotional support for patients before, nor the effect of putting on a uniform and having patients regard me as a professional.

> ### Over to you
>
> Summarise the learning that Melissa has identified from this incident.
> What other learning can you see in this account that she has not identified?
> Why might she not have seen this herself?

If you look closely at Figure 3.2, you will see that Melissa has not gone on to complete the final cue question posed by Johns, that of exploring the incident through what he has called 'ways of knowing'. This phrase relates back to the original purpose for his framework, to create a strategy for learning through uncovering the knowledge that we have and identifying what more we need to know in order to practise effectively. Johns is a nurse by background, and therefore has based his model in nursing. However, this provides a useful framework that is easily translated into other health-care professions, and therefore warrants further development here.

Johns considers it important to recognise our 'knowing' and has adopted a typology of knowledge identified by Barbara Carper in 1978. She identified four ways of knowing that can be found in nursing and named them:

- Empirics
- Ethics
- Personal
- Aesthetics.

**Empirics**  Carper calls this the science of nursing, which emerged as a concept in nursing during the late 1950s. It draws on traditional ideas of science in which reality is viewed as something that can be verified by other observers. Empirics are based on the assumption that what is known is that which is accessible through the senses, i.e. that can be observed and measured in some way. Empirics use the processes of describing, explaining and predicting the phenomena in the world through classic scientific methods. The ideal of scientific theory is that all its major ideas are expressed in terms that can be translated to 'out there' – empiric reality. Very often, theories of nursing, and other health-care professions, are seen to be lacking when judged against scientific parameters, and this was certainly the case when Carper was writing. What empirics give to us are the scientific background and theories that inform much of our practice. Examples of empirics that provide us with ways of knowing in health care are: physiological processes and anatomical structure; pharmacology; psychology etc.

**Ethics**  This incorporates what Carper called 'moral knowledge' or what is believed to be right or wrong in the way that we interact with other people. It includes matters of obligation or what ought to be done in particular situations. It involves making moment-to-moment judgements about what should be done, what is right and what is responsible. This may mean confronting conflicting values, norms, interests or principles in different situations. This is especially relevant for all kinds of professional health-care practice, as we are dealing with unique individuals over whom we very often have powers of life or death, and the quality of their lives. Our actions may determine the ways in which people experience their lives, particularly where they are unable to look after themselves, or make decisions that affect their lives – for instance, in the case of elderly people with dementia or people who are unconscious. Ethical knowing requires both an implicit knowing to base on-the-spot decisions on and knowledge of the formal principles and ethical theories of the disciplines. What it cannot do is to describe or predict what a decision should be; rather, it provides insight into what decisions are possible and why. The processes we use within our ethical knowing are those of clarifying, valuing and advocating for others.

**Personal knowing**  Carper sees this as the inner experience of becoming a whole, aware self. She suggests that, through knowing oneself, one is able to know another human being as a person because we have a concept of shared human experience. She says that we cannot reflect personal knowledge; that it is retrospective in that one can only describe the self that was when something was happening. The processes that we use in personal knowing are:

- Opening (being open to others)
- Centring (focusing on the patient)
- Realising (understanding the other person through recognising our own experiences).

**Aesthetics**  Carper sees this as the art of nursing, which involves seeing situations as wholes, not component parts. It is the way that nursing is expressed and made visible through actions, bearing, conduct, attitudes and the interactions of the nurse with her patients. She suggests that aesthetics involve what is possible, not necessarily what is concrete, as we reflect on alternative courses of action. This way of knowing includes what we learn as a result of our professional experiences. It is how we 'know' how to select from our total knowledge and wealth of experience that we have built up in the past, in order to perform what has been termed by Jacobs-Kramer and Chinn (1988) the 'art-act'. This is very often an unconscious process that we are not aware of unless we stop and think about it. The processes that we use in aesthetics are engaging, interpretation, envisioning.

Carper said that all four of these are present in all of our interactions, and that it is unlikely that one alone would inform the way that we act. However, they combine in different proportions, depending on what we are doing. While this approach to how we know the things that inform our professional actions arises from nursing, it is possible to use it to explore the ways that other health-care professions also use their sources of knowing. This is illustrated in the case study below.

## Case study

### Sue's experience – considering ways of knowing in a physiotherapy interaction

Sue is designing a rehabilitation programme for Mark, who injured his knee playing football. He has undergone surgery to the cruciate ligament in his left knee and now needs to work on rebuilding strength and mobility. The ways of knowing that inform her decisions can be broken down into Carper's framework as follows.

#### Empirics

Sue will use the information from her physical assessment of Mark to plan what exercises he will need and to predict a programme for his progress. These arise from her knowledge of anatomy and physiology and of healing processes. She will also draw on her ongoing physiotherapy education experiences, in which she learned a range of therapies and exercises that she can select from to design a programme appropriate to Mark's particular needs and that she can predict will be effective. She will also be taking into account Mark's age and lifestyle, what range of movement he would like to regain and what he will need to be able to do in the future. She also draws on her knowledge of motivational theories from psychology, and works within a cognitive framework of enabling Mark to understand the programme and what he is trying to achieve, so that he is committed to it as the best way forward for him.

#### Ethics

Sue's professional relationship with Mark is regulated by a professional code of conduct, by law and by the commonly accepted 'rules' of interpersonal relationships. He can expect her to treat him with respect and civility and to assure him that she has his best interests at heart. She needs to enable Mark to understand the programme

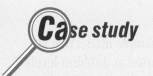

## Case study

### Robert's experience in the laboratory

#### What?

I work in the microbiology section of a hospital laboratory. I am responsible for overseeing the work of my section, as well as analysing and interpreting results from samples sent in. My particular specialty is wound swabs.

I had noticed, over a period of a few months, that the vast majority of swabs from geriatric inpatients result in MRSA being isolated.

#### So what?

If extended sensitivity tests are not set up on day 1 then there is a possible delay in the correct therapy being prescribed. Delays in correct treatment can be catastrophic for the patient concerned and can result in the spread of the organism to other patients. MRSA is becoming endemic in many hospital wards, particularly those for the elderly, and is a severe risk for vulnerable patients. However, the setting up of extra sensitivity tests where not needed is a waste of laboratory resources.

#### Now what?

For the benefit of the patient and all others, where *Staphylococcus aureus* is isolated from geriatric patients extended sensitivities should be set up on day 1.

This has now become common practice in the department.

#### Reflection on the use of the reflective framework

As a microbiologist working in a laboratory where our work is directed by standard operating procedures, I initially found it difficult to conceive of a situation where reflection could be useful. However, when I stepped back and thought about it more, I realised that it is easy to think about our work being simply about bench testing and experiments, and that there is actually a great deal going on beyond the world of the laboratory that influences and affects our work.

The incidence of MRSA in elderly patients had been increasing for months, yet, because the microbiologists had been dealing with the samples on an individual basis, the increase had gone unnoticed. It wasn't until I dealt with several in a row when covering for another member of staff that the penny dropped that there might be a problem here. Borton's framework enabled me to explore the situation rationally by using the cue questions. It is not complicated, and can be used with any type of situation. A more complicated framework would have put me off; many of these ask about feelings and personal action, which, to be quite honest, isn't appropriate in this sort of situation. The simple 'what–so what–now what' framework is easy to carry around in my head and use whenever a problem arises. I have even used it when dealing with other staff in a managerial capacity, and in helping to analyse problems within our multidisciplinary team in the lab.

Many students echo Robert's thoughts about the using Borton's framework. Its very simplicity means that it can be carried around in your head and easily remembered. Robert's example demonstrates the use of reflection to identify and solve problems, as opposed to dealing with a critical incident that may have arisen for an individual.

The difference between Borton's approach and Gibbs's and Johns's frameworks is clear in this example too, in that we can see that the reflective activity actually led to action being taken, rather than it being proposed or tentative. It moves from the realms of 'maybe' back into the real world of practice.

Borton's framework is being increasingly used by health-care professionals as a strategy for reflection, and this has prompted Rolfe *et al.* (2001) to develop it further in terms of adding in cue questions to flesh out the basic three questions. The expanded version is shown in Figure 3.4.

| Descriptive level of reflection | Theory and knowledge building level of reflection | Action-oriented level of reflection |
|---|---|---|
| **What** | **So what...** | **Now what...** |
| ... is the<br>• problem<br>• difficulty<br>• reason for being stuck<br>• reason for feeling bad<br>• reason we don't get on, etc.?<br>... was my role in the situation?<br>... was I trying to achieve?<br>... actions did I take?<br>... was the response of others?<br>... were the consequences:<br>• for my patient<br>• for myself<br>• for others?<br>... feelings did it invoke<br>• in the patients<br>• in myself<br>• in others?<br>... was good/bad about the experience? | ... does this tell me/teach me/imply/mean about:<br>• me<br>• my patient<br>• others<br>• our relationship<br>• my patient's care<br>• the model of care I am using<br>• my attitudes<br>• etc., etc.?<br>... was going through my mind as I acted?<br>... did I base my actions on?<br>... other knowledge can I bring to the situation?<br>... could/should I have done to make it better?<br>... is my new understanding of the situation?<br>... broader issues arise from the situation? | ... do I need to do in order to:<br>• make things better<br>• stop being stuck<br>• improve my patient's care<br>• resolve the situation<br>• feel better<br>• get on better<br>• etc., etc.?<br>... broader issues need to be considered if this action is to be successful?<br>... might be the consequences of this action? |

**Figure 3.4** *A framework for reflexive practice (Rolfe* et al. *2001)*

You will notice that this is called a framework for *reflexive*, as opposed to *reflective practice*. This means that the reflective spiral is created, as the action takes place in order to *change* the experience rather than simply to learn from it. The three key stages identified by Borton are built upon by incorporating the cyclical process described by Gibbs and many of the cue questions proposed by Johns. What makes the framework one for reflexive practice, is that action takes place as a result, and thus the experience is changed, producing a new situation. The reflexive practitioner therefore, is someone who continually practises reflectively, learning from and changing situations continually. This might seem a tall order when you are starting off as a student within a health-care profession. But, if you think about it, at some stage you will need to move into this way of practising, as you begin to make the links between the experiences that you have. You cannot go through life, or practice, simply having a series of unconnected experiences! Nor can you continue to explore your experiences only in the theoretical sense, as could happen if you only use Gibbs's model. By remaining in the theoretical stages of reflection, all you will do is identify your learning using reflective processes, you will not be a reflective practitioner, nor will you be practising reflexively.

Borton's framework is a generic one that can be used by anyone, and indeed, Rolfe *et al.* (2001) provide two issues to be considered before it is adopted, suggesting that active selection is needed. They suggest:

- They are presenting a framework, not a model, making no claims that it is a representation or description of the process of reflection; it is merely an ordered set of cues through which the practitioner might structure reflective thoughts.

- It is a generic framework that can be employed to structure internal, spoken, or written reflections either alone, with a facilitator, or in a group. Because of this it may not suit individual needs, and the cue questions are therefore intended to be open to change and revision for different practitioners in different situations.

## Reflective activity

Try using Borton's framework for yourself. You could choose either the simplified 'what – so what – now what' version, or work through the expanded one proposed by Rolfe *et al*.

It is worth taking some time in choosing the experience to reflect on. You could re-work the previous example that you used in the Gibbs or Johns frameworks. If you do this you'll have a comparison of what you learned from both, and be able to evaluate how useful each of them will be to you. Alternatively, you may choose to select a completely different experience or incident.

Work through the different stages to complete the reflective process.
Once you have done that, take a few minutes to evaluate the framework itself.

- How useful did you find Borton's or Rolfe *et al*.'s framework?
- How easy was it to use?
- Did you have any difficulties using it?
- Did it enable you to see the event from a wider perspective?
- Did it enable you to reach alternative conclusions about the event to the ones you had when you started out?
- Did it help you to frame action that you could take?
- Did you take the action?
- How comfortable did you feeling using it?
- Would you choose to use it again?

Try to give the reasons for your answers to these questions.

Of course, what we also see in using Borton's framework is the beginnings of the reflective spiral. If you take the action that you have identified, it presents you with a continuation of the event, and thus more to reflect on! Many students use this continual spiral to develop deeper and deeper understanding of situations. This is very effective if you are engaged in problem-based learning and need to keep a record of how you gain more knowledge and where it comes from. This can then be used to predict your actions, try them out and reflect further on how your practice has changed as a result of your increased understanding.

**Key points** Top tips

- Borton's framework leads through the ERA reflective stages completely; hence action is taken as a result of the reflective activity
- Borton's framework has the simple cue questions of What?, So what? and Now what?
- It is relatively easy to use

**Over to you**

The choice of which framework to use for your reflective activity is clearly a choice for you. However, it is worth taking the time to consider why you would select a particular framework, so that you make a conscious decision.
Look back over the critical incidents you have explored using the three models in this chapter.

- Which model did you feel most comfortable using?
- Why was this?
- Would you choose to use this model all the time?
- What are the differences between the models?
- Can you imagine any situations where you would choose to use the different models?
- Would you want to adapt or change them in any ways to suit your particular situations?

## Conclusions

In this chapter you have met three different frameworks for reflection that you can choose to use in your own reflective activities. You will come across others, and may well be given alternatives as part of your own course. The purpose of selecting these three was to provide you with alternatives that have arisen from different disciplines, from different standpoints and for different purposes. All of these are sufficiently flexible to enable you to develop them to suit your own needs. You can, of course, choose to adapt them by adding or leaving out components. You might also find that you create your own framework when you are sufficiently confident at working with the principles of reflection to be able to do so.

If you have been working through the activities in this chapter, you will have created three 'model' cases, each using one of the frameworks that we have presented to you. Each of these will have used a critical incident, so you have also got a clearer understanding of what it means to learn from your own experiences.

Each of these strategies can help us in the quest for developing and changing our practice. Without a doubt, equally useful in achieving this is the act of exploring our own critical incidents. This enables us to build our understanding of our own practice, and to develop our knowledge on the basis of needs that we identify for ourselves.

Finally, the cue to action that arises from engaging in reflective practice is itself a step towards developing our own clinical practice. Each can be used within a variety of reflective situations, and are flexible enough to be used both by yourself and with others

---

### RRRRRRapid recap

Check your progress so far by working through each of the following questions.

1. What are Goodman's three levels of reflection?
2. What are the six stages of Gibbs's reflective cycle?
3. What might be a drawback to using Gibbs's cycle within reflective practice?
4. What are the main differences between Gibbs's and Johns's frameworks?
5. What are Carper's types of knowing?
6. What are Borton's three cue questions?

If you have difficulty with more than one of the questions, read through the section again to refresh your understanding before moving on.

---

## References

Borton, T. (1970) *Reach, Touch and Teach*. London: Hutchinson.

Carper, B. (1978) Fundamental patterns of knowing in nursing. *Advances in Nursing Science*, **1**, 13–23.

Gibbs, G. (1988) *Learning by Doing: A guide to teaching and learning methods*. Further Education Unit, Oxford Polytechnic, Oxford.

Goodman, J. (1984) Reflection and teacher education: a case study and theoretical analysis. *Interchanges*, **15**, 9–26.

Jacobs-Kramer, M.K. and Chinn, P.L. (1988) Perspectives on knowing: a model of nursing knowledge. *Scholarly Inquiry for Nursing Practice*, **2**, 129–139.

Johns, C. (1998) Opening the doors of perception, in *Transforming Nursing Through Reflective Practice* (eds C. Johns and D. Freshwater), pp. 1–20. Blackwell Science, Oxford.

Johns, C. (2000) *Becoming a Reflective Practitioner*. Blackwell Science, Oxford.

Palmer, A., Burns, S. and Bulman, C. (1994) *Reflective Practice in Nursing*. Blackwell Scientific Publications, Oxford.

Rolfe, G., Freshwater, D. and Jasper, M. (2001) *Critical Reflection for Nursing and the Helping Professions: A user's guide*. Palgrave, Basingstoke.

# 4

# Entering the clinical environment

In this chapter you will be thinking about the challenges you may meet when entering the clinical environment, and how, by anticipating and acknowledging your feelings, worries and anxieties through reflection, you are likely to be more prepared for what you might encounter. The chapter will establish the differing nature of the relationships that you will encounter in the clinical environment. In particular, it will examine the tensions you will meet in being a student within a workplace, in encountering situations you are not prepared for, which might be unexpected, and in managing unfamiliar situations by drawing on your previous experiences.

Hopefully, this will be a gentle introduction and preparation for going into the clinical environment and encountering real life situations in practice.

An essential difference between college and your placements is that you will be entering a world whose primary function is to deliver a service to its patients. While you are there to learn, and to learn through observing and providing care under supervision, the others you encounter are there essentially to provide care. Part of their role may be to support learners in the environment, but others you meet will not have a teaching or support component to their job, and although they will recognise you as a student, they are more likely to consider you as simply another worker. This will be especially so of the patients, or clients, that you meet. So, although you know you are a student, many others will not and will have different expectations of you from the ones you have of yourself. It is important, therefore, to think carefully about your role as a student when you go into different clinical settings, not only to get the most out of the experiences they can offer you but also in terms of:

- The relationships you have with others
- Your status within the clinical environment
- The responsibilities that you have as a student practitioner
- What you need to learn from your placements.

## Identifying your role as a student in the clinical environment

Initially, entering clinical areas as a student can be very daunting and you will probably experience feelings of anxiety many times as you change placements in order to build up your repertoire of experiences and skills from different settings. No matter what your previous experiences are of working in clinical environments, when you re-enter as a student your role will be different. You are there primarily to learn. While this learning may occur from actively working in the area or from specific learning opportunities that are arranged for you, it is your responsibility, working together with your supervisor, to ensure that you achieve the learning that the placement has to offer. In order to maximise your learning from placements it is worth taking some time to think about your role as a student in the clinical environment, so that you can plan to achieve what you need to from it.

### Reflective activity

The nature of learning in college and from work placements is very different, as is your role in each one. Try to work through the following questions, either by yourself or with another person, and consider how you can use the different learning environments most effectively to fulfil your learning needs.

- What are the differences between college and the clinical arena as learning environments?
- What opportunities for learning will be available in the clinical environment?
- What will the clinical areas give you that you cannot get from college?
- What is your role in the clinical environment?
- What responsibilities do you have as a student within the clinical environment in relation to:
  - Yourself
  - The patients and their carers
  - The staff with whom you will be working
- Who is available to provide you with support in these environments?
- What else can provide you with guidance while in the clinical areas?

This is what Carrie decided to do.

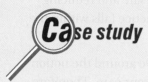
**Case study**

I politely told Lisa that I had been taught not to lift patients as there was a great risk of hurting myself, the other lifter and the patient. I went for the sling hoist, which was just outside the bathroom, and together Lisa and I used it to assist Jim into the wheelchair. I told Jim to stay calm, and went to get the nurse. Lisa said that there was no need as it was only a minor slip, but I told her that we could never be sure so it was safe to let a qualified member of staff know. I then went and explained the situation to my mentor, who came with me to the bathroom to assess Jim and the state of his leg.

---

**Reflective activity**

What were Carrie's responsibilities to Lisa when she was working with her?
If you were in this position, what would be going through your mind in terms of your feelings, and your role as a student?
What, in terms of your knowledge and previous experience, can you use to make sense of this situation?

---

This is how Carrie reflected on, and learned from, the experience.

Heavy lifting causes accidents in the workplace such as back pain and injury. The Health and Safety Executive (1998) reported over 15 000 manual handling accidents in the health-care sector and, of these, over 60% were related to patient handling. Accordingly, all health-care organisations must have a Manual Handling policy to benefit both patients and staff. Safe handling often adds up to the quality of care that a patient receives. A safe handling policy also reduces accidents as well as sick leave for the staff (Pheasant 1998). The Royal College of Nursing (2002) developed a code of practice for handling patients that specified that two nurses should lift no more than 50.8kg. I refused to lift Jim because I knew it was wrong according to the Manual Handling policy of the hospital. It was not right for Jim and certainly not right for us as well. I therefore feel that my actions were in everyone's best interests. If we had lifted Jim we might have caused further damage to him, and injured our backs. On reflection, Lisa might have wanted to lift Jim manually because of lack of training, which meant she was unable to identify the risk, or it could just have been to save time as a result of the low staffing levels. Her actions could also have resulted from lack of communication and inadequate information about Jim at handover, which resulted in assumptions about his capabilities.

At the time the incident was happening I felt angry at Lisa, who, after working in the hospital for 10 years had failed to adhere to the Manual Handling policy. I also thought she was taking advantage of me as a student, who she thought would agree to do as she was told. When she asked me to lift Jim I felt I had to advocate for Jim as he had been shocked by the whole event and was unable to speak for himself. My actions were influenced by what I had been taught in class with regard to manual handling and risk assessments. At the back of my mind I could hear the lecturer saying 'Tell them politely that you cannot do it as it is wrong', which I did. I also knew that Jim could not put weight on his right leg because of his hip.

I later had a discussion with my mentor and pointed out that some ward staff had probably done their Manual Handling courses a long time ago and hence needed to be updated with the new policies. She said she would see to it that everyone went on a short course to update their certificates.

I feel, on reflection, that I did the right thing here. I am pleased that none of us were hurt as a result of the incident. Reflecting on this incident has helped me to apply theory to practice, and work according to the code of professional conduct that states that people in the nursing profession should act in such a manner as to safeguard and promote the well being of patients and others (Nursing and Midwifery Council 2002). My assertiveness skills were enhanced as I managed to stand my ground by refusing to do what I felt was wrong. I have realised that I can learn from immediate personal experiences in practice. The incident has been a valuable learning experience as I have learned at first hand how to use theories of reflection, and it has encouraged me to think more critically about the ability to use theory in practice. I have also realised that, even though I am a new student, I still have responsibilities to others, even if they are older than me and have more experience.

I do hope that the staff get the updating that they need and that lifting practices change as a result.

### References

Health and Safety Executive (1998) *Manual Handling Operations: Guidance on the regulations*, 2nd edn. HSE, London.

Nursing and Midwifery Council (2002) *Code of Professional Conduct*. NMC, London.

Pheasant, S. (1998) *Manual Handling: An ergonomic approach*. National Backpain Association, Teddington.

Royal College of Nursing (2002) *Changing Practice – Improving Health: An integrated back injury prevention programme for nursing and care homes*. RCN, London.

---

**Key points**   *Top tips*

- Remember that you are primarily a student and are placed in practice for the specific purpose of learning from that environment
- Practice placements are working environments – their primary purpose is to deliver care, you will be expected to fit in with the other people there, not the other way round!
- You have responsibilities to the patients and their carers, to other staff and colleagues and to yourself – these are all equally important
- It is normal to experience 'reality shock', anxiety and insecurity when entering new environments; these can be used positively to focus you on what you need to achieve from the experiences available in the placement

---

Carrie draws attention to the need for assertiveness skills, especially when faced with people attempting to exert their authority over you. Part of your role in clinical environments will be to act independently and to ensure that you can justify and defend your behaviour and actions at all times. Often this means developing other skills as a student that will carry you forward into self-regulated professional practice. As Carrie has started to be, you will need to be self-empowered as a student to maximise your learning in clinical placements.

## Self-empowerment

So much of what you do during your course is directed by the need to qualify, such as satisfying the professional bodies, completing the specified competencies and achieving the learning outcomes for the course, that it is easy to feel that you have little control yourself as a student.

However, do remember that these outcomes are provided for you as defined endpoints in the course, and the means to achieve them will be offered to you. But it is how you plan to use these, and the attitude you take towards using the experiences on offer within your clinical placements, that will determine how much you achieve from the breadth of pre-qualifying experiences you have. Taking the opportunities to empower yourself is as much a part of your course as all of the other components.

The reflective cycle provides you with a mechanism for self-empowerment, and the positive reinforcement that you get from being able to take control of your learning will be important to you in feeling that you are part of your own destiny.

Consider Josie's approach to her clinical placement in the following case study.

We can see how Josie has used the ERA reflective cycle effectively here to plan to get the most from her new placement.

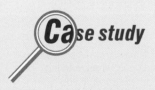
**Case study**

### Josie's forward planning

As Josie turned off her light to go to sleep, she was quietly satisfied with her preparations for her new placement, starting the next day. She was looking forward to her placement with the Community Occupational Therapist based in the Social Services Department. Having already completed 2 years of her course and a range of hospital placements, the next few months were going to be spent in the community experiencing the different working needs and demands of visiting people in their own homes and in residential settings. She even had an alternative placement arranged in America, where she would be visiting a rehabilitation hospital for burns victims.

*Case study continued*

Josie had taken the time to work out what she needed to ach
placement, in terms of both her overall needs for skills required for her j
and the course work she had to complete by the end of the semester. She planned
to evaluate and compare the assessment schedules from her last placement with
the one used in the community as one assignment. And wanting to focus her
dissertation on the specific needs of young, spinally injured patients retraining for
new careers, she had liaised with her new supervisor to spend time with the
Occupational Therapist in the local residential unit.

She was confident that she would get on well with Jane, her community supervisor,
as she had spoken to her on the phone already and they had talked about the
competencies that she needed to achieve from this placement. As a result, she knew
that Jane had planned a schedule of visits, both by herself and with other members
of staff, to give her the experiences that she needed. She had also mentioned her
assignments and assessment schedule, so that Jane would be aware of what she
was doing in her study time and could look out for anything happening that would
help with those. Finally, Josie had worked out a rough time plan for getting the work
completed this semester so that she wouldn't feel under too much pressure. Her bag
was packed for tomorrow and she had made sure that she had her competencies
and assessment documents with her so that she and Jane could really put their first
morning together to good use. Time was going so fast now, with finals looming,
and she felt that she couldn't afford to miss any opportunities to get closer to fulfilling
the packed schedule of the last 9 months of the course. As she went to sleep that
night she was confident that she had done all that she could to get the most out
of this placement.

The *event* itself was to be the upcoming placement in the
community. The stages of the reflective cycle can be broken down and
applied in the following way.

**Stage 1: Identifying the experience/critical incident**  Josie started from
the point of identifying what it was that she needed to achieve by
looking at her assessment schedule, her competency document and
the opportunities that would be available in the community. She was
also anticipating her needs following that in terms of her elective
placement and her dissertation.

**Stage 2: Observing and describing the experience**  From these Josie
was able to anticipate what it was she wanted to achieve from the
clinical placement. These she had phrased as learning needs that
matched her outcomes. She was able to predict what opportunities
would be available in her new placement.

**Stage 3: Analysing the experience**  She was then able to break down
the opportunities available, on the basis of her previous knowledge and
experience and what she had been told by her lecturers, her new
supervisor and her student colleagues, and match these to her
learning needs.

**Stage 4: Interpreting the experience**  From the experience available within the clinical placement she was able to select what was appropriate and most likely to enable her to achieve what she wanted. She also realised that there were unknowns that would be encountered, and that these would add to the breadth of her experiences.

**Stage 5: Exploring alternatives**  Having realised that there were competencies that she needed to develop but were not already planned by her supervisor, she explored other ways of getting these. This included asking Jane if she could spend extended time at the spinal injuries intermediate care unit to gather information for her dissertation. She also wanted to apportion her time so that she could complete the comparative assignment on OT assessment from the examples she found in the community. All of these meant that she was making the most of the opportunities that might be available, and gearing them specifically to her own learning needs.

**Stage 6: Framing action**  Josie planned to phone Jane to ensure that her perceptions and ideas were on the right lines. She was also anxious about the first meeting with Jane and wanted to know what she sounded like to allay her fears. She planned an assessment schedule to complete her assignments for this semester on time in order to take the pressure off and know that she was planning to complete her work by the submission dates. She provisionally ticked off the competencies for this placement, and also those that came from other sections, in her book so she knew she hadn't overlooked anything.

Finally, Josie completed the ERA cycle by carrying out the action that she had planned. She had spoken to Jane and ensured that she knew when and where she was expected the following day. She had packed her bag and ensured that she had the documents with her that she needed. Her time plan and work schedule were on her wall. She knew what she hoped to achieve during the placement, and was content that there was not much more she could have done in preparation.

Josie might appear to be the 'model' student, yet all that she had done was to choose to spend a couple of hours in reflection and forward planning. As a result she did achieve her required competencies, her assignments and the extra things that she had wanted to get from the experience. Her deliberate use of time in reflection in this way actually saved her time overall, as she wasn't wasting her energy worrying about not having enough time or having to catch up with things that could have been planned in advance.

Contrast this with Justin's approach, in the following case study.

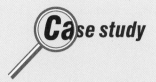

### Justin lives for the moment

'So, what is it that you need to achieve from your placement in Intensive Care then, Justin?' asked Kerrie.

'Er... well, I haven't really thought about it. Until I see what you do and what goes on here, I won't know, will I?' replied Justin.

'OK, so let's think about your assignments, then, and your competencies for this semester. What college work do you have to do that we can tie in with your placement here?' said Kerrie, hoping that this might provide a focus for what was turning out to be a difficult first meeting with her student.

'I don't know. I think we may have an ethics assignment, and I suppose I need to start thinking about a dissertation topic. But to be quite honest, I don't have a clue,' replied Justin.

'Well, think about that and we'll talk about it later in the week. Now, your competencies – let's see what else you have left to cover and what we need to plan to include in your time here.'

'Um... well, I haven't got it with me, I forgot it in the rush to get out this morning. Had a late night with the boys last night and didn't get much sleep. You know how it goes....'

In fact, Justin is a classic case of a student who thinks that life simply happens – and that his failure to get work in on time, get good marks, achieve his competencies and find his course interesting has nothing to do with him. As a result, he considered himself to be disorganised and a failure, and envied others who appeared to sail through life with no problems. He had a record of late submissions, not knowing where he was going, turning up to placements late and misunderstanding what work needed to be done. Consequently, despite being a likeable and personable student, his tutors and clinical assessors doubted that he had the attitude or strength of character to act responsibly and independently as a professional practitioner. He lacked neither academic nor clinical ability, but he was totally oblivious to the fact that all these things were under his control. He couldn't see that, in failing to assess and plan his course, he was not developing the independence and organisational capacities that would be expected of him when qualified and responsible and accountable for his own actions, and those of others.

> ## *Over to you*
>
> Take some time to think about your usual approach to starting a new placement. Are you a Josie or a Justin?
>
> While these students represent the two extremes of behaviour, it is likely that you recognise some of these characteristics in yourself. For instance:
>
> - Do you forward plan when going into new situations?
> - Do you identify your goals and what you want to achieve?
> - Do you set yourself time schedules?
> - Do you blame other people for things that go wrong in your life?
> - Do you see things as beyond your control – such as not having enough time to do things?
> - Do you feel sometimes that you are lacking in ability, and that this is why you don't get good marks, or fail exams?
>
> What can you learn from your answers to these questions?
>
> Do you need to change your behaviour in any way so that you can plan to achieve what you want to, rather than less, as you often do through failing to plan?

This section has been about empowering yourself as a student. Empowerment is about taking responsibility for our own actions. Empowerment as a student is about enabling yourself to achieve what you need to for the future. To be empowered, we need sufficient information on which to make decisions and the drive to plan on the basis of that information. Perhaps more importantly, though, is that we need to believe in ourselves, in our own capacity and ability to achieve what we want to. We need to adopt an attitude that says 'I can and I will'. One way to do this is to plan for the future and be determined to carry out those plans. Who do you think will be successful in their lives – Josie or Justin? Can you identify your reasons for thinking this?

## Identifying learning experiences in the clinical environment

Within reflective practice the experiences that you have are used as the foundations for actively, and consciously, learning in a professional capacity. Throughout your professional education, and in all of the placements that you gain practical experience, you will build up a range of different situations and examples that provide the foundations of your professional knowledge. While it is impossible to reflect actively on all of these, it is the conscious reflection on some of them that will enable you to capitalise on what you are doing and recognise that you are learning as you progress through your course. In a way, reflective practice is a short cut to learning. You will learn more quickly if you get into the habit of reflecting on your experiences, identifying the learning that you have achieved and the action that you need to take as a result.

## Reflective activity

### Why do you do what you do?

It is worth taking the time to think about the different opportunities and sources of experience that may arise from the clinical environment. Take a few minutes to reflect on the nature of the clinical environment. Identify the types of experience and situation you may encounter that will provide opportunities for learning. For instance:

- What ways do you use to learn in the college setting?
- How will learning in the clinical environment differ from learning in a college setting?
- What things can you do to ensure that you learn in these environments?
- What can you do to ensure that you recognise your learning?
- How can you use other people to help you learn in clinical environments?
- What responsibilities do you have for organising your learning in the clinical environment?
- What is available to help and guide you in identifying and organising these responsibilities?

There are different ways that we can think about these opportunities, and many of these will have been included in your list.

## Learning from others

As a student you will always be working under the supervision of a qualified member of staff, and will meet other professionals in the course of your experiences. You will also meet many other people in different professions, as clients and carers, as users of health-care services and as colleagues and co-workers in support services. These each offer different opportunities for learning.

### Your supervisor

Initially, it is primarily from your supervisor that you will be learning, as you use them as a role model for the way that you act in the clinical environment. Together you will work on identifying what it is you need to learn and on planning your experiences so that you have the opportunities to achieve these goals. The relationship between yourself and your supervisor is a relatively formal one, as it may be the supervisor who assesses your progress and competence. The supervisor is also ultimately responsible for you while you are in the workplace and is accountable for the actions that you undertake under their professional supervision. They need to ascertain your capabilities for themselves before trusting you to take responsibility with patients. Therefore, it is here that you are likely to be able to gain structure in planning your experiences in the clinical environment, and work towards meeting planned goals and objectives through your supervisor's guidance and support. Your supervisor will be your first contact in the placement and the initial person you will turn to throughout the time you spend in the area. Your supervisor is also likely to be the lynchpin around which the whole placement revolves, as they know the area, the types of opportunities available and the specific strengths and skills of other members of staff.

### Other qualified staff and students in your own professional field

You will, of course, work with many others in your own clinical speciality. This might happen in a formal or informal way. For instance, another practitioner may have been asked to work with you for the day because they have particular expertise or are going to visit a certain client who offers you experience of certain conditions that you might not get with your supervisor. This is particularly the case where practitioners hold their own caseloads and have built up experience over many years in one area of practice. Your supervisor may decide that others can offer you a wider range of experiences in this way than they can themselves. In addition, you will have many opportunities for discussion with your own colleagues.

Working with others in your own chosen profession, whether they are your supervisors or other qualified staff, enables you to learn, and take on, the attributes of being a practitioner in this particular profession – we call these socialisation processes.

These socialisation processes enable you to function within your own professional world. They include becoming familiar with the language, ways of working, attitudes, skills and professional attributes that go along with your profession. It is almost impossible to acquire these without working with others. It is similar to learning the rules of a game in order to win. You learn these by observing and mimicking the ways in which your role models conduct themselves as practitioners. In this way, you will build up the attributes that make you acceptable to others in your profession; and other attributes will become extinct. You may find that you admire and respect some people more than others and deliberately try to adopt the ways in which they work. Other people may not impress you so much and you may catch yourself making a mental note not to emulate their behaviour. Use your experiences of working with others in your field as a focus for reflection. This will enable you to work on becoming the type of practitioner who exhibits these features, so that you become recognisable as a member of that profession. You will also find that you become more comfortable with others as a result, as you start to display those attributes yourself and fit in with the others around you.

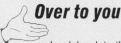

### Over to you

Look back to the reflective activity on professional attributes in Chapter 2.

Your answers to the last three questions in this activity will have begun to clarify for you the type of image that you admire in a practitioner. They will have started to set standards for you to achieve as you develop and acquire an identity as one of those practitioners yourself. In learning about professional practice, we tend to unconsciously emulate those around us with whom we can identify. In doing this exercise, you will now be more aware of the characteristics and attributes of others that you can consciously make a note of and consider in light of your own development and behaviour. An example of how this happened to one student nurse is described in the following case study, an account written by a student nurse.

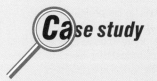

### Case study

### Witnessing unprofessional behaviour

The incident took place in the ward office during handover. A 15-year-old girl, Anne, had been admitted to the ward 2 days before to have a lump removed from her left leg. She was also 6 months pregnant. Her mum, Mrs West, had been very worried about her and was constantly by her side during visiting times. The day Anne had her operation she was in a lot of pain and her mum wanted to stay with her all night. The night staff did not permit her to do so as it was against hospital regulations. Mrs West was, however, assured that her daughter would be well cared for and that she would be contacted if the need arose. She did not like the arrangement and became abusive, but left eventually and returned early the next morning.

During handover, Sister Molly said:

'Oh, that Mrs West and her daughter are trouble makers! The mum didn't want to leave last night and made so much noise about it. Anyway, it's not as if her daughter is the first to have an operation, and it's certainly not our fault that she is pregnant at 15. Watch out for them.'

She then went on to say that Anne needed a 'motherectomy' because of the attitude and behaviour of her mother. Molly was saying all this without realising that the door was not fully closed and that Mrs West happened to be passing by just then. Mrs West heard everything that was said.

Everyone in the office froze with fright and embarrassment. It was agreed that Molly should apologise but she refused to do so as she felt she had told the truth.

Reflect *Reflective activity*

What are your initial reactions to this incident?

How would you have felt if you had been a witness?

What are your impressions about the behaviour of the ward sister in:

- Saying what she said in handover in the first place?
- Refusing to apologise to the patient?

**The student involved continued her account.**

I felt so offended and disgusted about the whole incident. I could not understand how Molly could speak about human beings, people for whom we were meant to be caring, in this way. While the Sister may have tried some irreverent humour, which many nurses do in isolation because of the pressures of the job, by saying 'motherectomy', this went beyond humour. I would have found this surprising in itself, coming from someone with her status and authority, but to have it witnessed by the person she was referring to was just awful. The whole episode was a culture shock for me, especially as it was said during a handover, which is meant to be a factual presentation of the patients between shifts. A handover is a powerful medium, as information shared at that time stays with us for the rest of the shift. If someone is described in a certain way, it can sometimes be difficult to step aside from that description and really assess a person on their own qualities; thus patients become labelled, and it is difficult as the practitioner to put that aside once it has been heard. I really felt that what the Sister had said was very unfair because she was forming an opinion for all of us based on her feelings.

While Molly may have felt that she had only said what had happened, the manner in which she did it was not professional at all. It is important as health professionals to always show cultural sensitivity, respect equality and be open-minded. Although it was right for Molly to relay information to us, it was not right for her to be judgemental and express her personal opinions. Thompson *et al.* (1984) suggest that the manner in which information and confidences are shared is a sensitive indicator of whether professional attitudes are creating dependency or whether they are used to assist patients towards autonomy and help them take control of their own lives. This means that, if the handover information had been said as if Anne and her mother were present, no one would have been hurt, the Sister would not have looked unprofessional and the rest of the staff would not have been so embarrassed. Molly's actions show that she was not acting in the best interests of the patient and her carers. Thompson *et al.* go on to say that, as professionals, treating people as unique individuals involves respecting their rights at all times. In this case, the fact that Anne was pregnant should not have been an issue for Molly, it was nothing to do with the reason that she had been admitted. While Mrs West might have been a nuisance to the ward staff, her behaviour was out of concern for her daughter – being treated with care and consideration by the nursing staff would have helped to allay her anxieties and made the experience a more positive one for both of them. By showing such negative feelings towards Anne and her mother, Molly showed a lack of pastoral care and empathy.

The impression that Anne and her mother have of nurses is that they gossip and are untrustworthy. If Molly had apologised for what she had said, this might have been rectified. But she compounded the problem by refusing to say sorry for what she had said.

**References**

Thompson, I.E., Melia, K.M. and Boyd, K.M. (1994) *Nursing Ethics*, 3rd edn. Churchill Livingstone, Edinburgh.

---

### Reflective activity

What have you learned from this case study about the responsibilities that we have as professionals when referring to patients? How do you feel about the ward sister's refusal to apologise?

What are the differences between the ways in which we refer to others when we are acting in a professional capacity and the sorts of thing we can say in private?

Are there any implications arising from your code of professional conduct that you might refer to here?

What impressions might the public gain, from incidents like this, about the ways in which professionals act?

In terms of your own future behaviour, what decisions can you take now about the ways in which you will talk about your patients to other people when acting in a professional capacity?

---

This is how the student concerned summarised her learning.

I have learned that privacy is of the utmost importance during handovers in order to protect information shared during that time. Personal feelings should not interfere with handovers, and we should not give our opinions about other people, whether we approve of their behaviour or not. We should instead concentrate on factual information and patients' needs for care. I would apologise if I offended a patient in any way.

I have also learned that there are boundaries between our role as a professional and our role as a private person. In nursing, because we are with patients for extended periods of time, it is easy to slip into being friendly and maybe muddying the differences between how we would act as a professional and how we would act as a friend. It is important for me to develop professional ways of relating to people, and I have learned here that it is very easy to cross those boundaries. I will be careful to keep my personal views about people to myself, or perhaps to only share them when I am away from the clinical area, where I can give my viewpoints, rather than being in a professional working relationship.

I now also appreciate how important recognising good role models will be for my development. This incident was a crucial one for me as it was so extreme. I had heard other nurses hand over before and say things like 'He's a lovely gentleman' or 'He's a dirty old man' and really thought nothing of it. But this incident has really brought it home to me how inappropriate it is to make personal remarks about anyone. I think the rule of never saying anything about anyone that you wouldn't say in front of them is a really good one, and one that I will try to always observe in the future.

*Case study continued*

I have gained much from reflecting on this incident. The structured process has intensified my self-awareness and made me analyse the extent to which my own thoughts, feelings and actions can affect the provision of quality nursing care. Reflection has been a good learning experience for me and is certainly a tool I will use throughout my practice to identify areas of practice that I think are in need of further development, and those areas that may already have been successfully developed.

## Qualified staff and students in other professional fields

Similarly, in today's multidisciplinary health-care world, you will always be encountering practitioners and students from other professions. These people will provide you with differing perspectives on caring for others from those that come from your own profession.

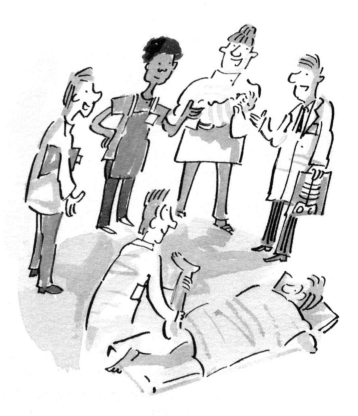

*Working with many different health-care professions enriches your professional development*

## Over to you

Take some time now to think about the features of some of the different health-care professions that you have met.

First, write down the features of your own profession. For instance, think about:

● What it was that attracted you to this profession instead of others
● The key features of your profession, i.e. what distinguishes you from other health-care workers
● What type of care you provide to patients
● The environment in which you provide that care
● The nature of the relationship you have with patients
● The type of education that prepares practitioners
● The relationships you have with other professional groups
● The degree of independence your profession has within the health-care field

Now, using the same identifying features, compare these with at least two other professional groups. Those you might choose from are:

● Nurses
● Midwives
● Physiotherapists
● Occupational therapists
● Radiographers
● Social workers
● Operating department practitioners
● Doctors
● Clinical psychologists
● Dietitians

Finally, think about what you could learn from these other groups that will help your own development as a practitioner. How can these groups complement the care that you provide for patients? If you had the opportunity to spend time with people from these professions, what is it that you would want to gain from that experience?

Making the most of the experience of other people is important for you in developing your own skills. Very few practitioners work in isolation in caring for patients. You will increasingly find yourself attending team meetings and discussions involving a range of workers from different disciplines, all of whom provide their own perspective on caring for the patient they are focussing on. It is by understanding the parameters within which these professionals work, and the areas of expertise and responsibility that they have, that you will come to develop a deeper understanding of your own role. But you will also learn to appreciate the alternative skills and perspectives that others

**Keywords**

**Paradigm cases**
Separate cases that we build up as a repertoire of experience and use to reflect back to when we meet similar experiences again.

**Key points** Top tips

- Identify the other people in each placement that can help you to achieve your learning needs
- Develop a working relationship with your supervisor that focuses on what you need to get from the placement
- Remember that your supervisor is also likely to be your assessor and is a practitioner in their own right, with roles and responsibilities defined by codes of professional conduct and the supervisor's contract of employment
- Other qualified practitioners in your own field, and from other disciplines, have a wealth of experience that they are willing to share – try to capitalise on this when planning your learning and experiences
- Remember that we have responsibilities to our patients, co-workers and other students – we may have more information and knowledge than they do

bring to problems and situations, which will broaden your understanding of working within a multidisciplinary workforce.

While learning from working with other people is very important, you will also find that you can learn from what is going on around you, in terms of the opportunities available in the specific clinical context of your placement.

## Learning from clinical placements

During your course your clinical placements will be selected to ensure that you have the opportunities to experience a broad range of health-care settings and contexts. Each one offers different experiences for you to develop knowledge, skills and competencies contributing to your overall development as a practitioner. Over the length of your course, it is likely that you will only visit each specialty once, and therefore it is very important that you plan to gain as much from the placement as it has to offer.

At other times you may experience client attachment or caseload allocation. These offer a different sort of experience, where you learn through building up your experiences by assessing, planning and providing care. These types of placements offer the experience of relatively long-term interactions with patients, where you follow a person through their encounter with your particular service, and therefore you build up your own bank of **paradigm cases** from which to draw on later in your professional life.

Your placements will be divided into mainstream placements, which will help you to build the essential characteristics of your own profession, and alternative placements, which offer you extra experiences during which you also learn your role. These may be dependent on your own interests within a particular field and on the types of opportunity available. Many courses offer optional or elective placements where students are able to choose where they go; some may even be in a different country or health-care system, in a different

---

### Reflective activity

Take some time now to think about the types of experience offered during your course. Even if you only know your placements for a few months, or the first year, you can still reflect on the learning that you will be able to achieve from them.

● How many of these placements are designed to provide you with the core knowledge, skills and experience that characterise your profession?

● What are these placements?

● What other placements will you be experiencing?

● How will these supplement your learning from your core placements?

What do you think is the purpose of these placements?

---

part of the country or specialty, or in specialist clinical areas that develop skills not normally expected in pre-qualifying experience.

Of course, the many professional groups involved in health-care delivery mean that each professional group has a different way of organising care, and therefore can offer different types of experience. For instance, operating department practitioners (ODPs) have very specific roles in working with patients who are undergoing surgical procedures. However, this activity may not be confined to operating theatres alone. Anywhere that an anaesthetic is being administered and patients need to be cared for while under its influence may be seen as offering experience for students. So, outpatient clinics where patients undergo minor procedures, or X-ray departments where investigations are done, may also be offering clinical placements for student ODPs. Similarly, the student ODP needs to know what happens to patients before they get to the operating department, in terms of preparation for their operation. This is particularly important where complicated surgery will be taking place, or where surgery may have long term consequences. So a student ODP may also be offered short-term placements in an intensive care unit or on a general surgical ward in order to develop their perspective of their own specialty. This enables the student to place their care within the context of care delivered by the other professional disciplines. The following case study shows how one ODP student broadened his perspective of caring for patients while in an observational placement.

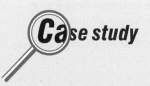

## Seeing the whole person

During the night Mrs Jones, a 78-year-old lady, was admitted to the ward with a fractured left wrist following a fall. She also had multi-infarct dementia and lived in a nursing home. She was classified as nil-by-mouth on arrival in anticipation of corrective surgery. At 14.30 a nurse and I took Mrs Jones to the trauma room in A&E as the fractured wrist was to be treated conservatively (without surgery). The doctor was to manipulate the bone back into the correct position, thus reducing the fracture, after which the wrist would be immobilised in a back slab plaster. The procedure was to be done under a general anaesthetic and so the doctor hadn't administered morphine before moving her from the ward as it wouldn't be necessary and, as a respiratory depressant, would be a risk for Mrs Jones. When we arrived, however, he said that he would use a local anaesthetic after all. The nurse suggested that Mrs Jones was given morphine and that the procedure was delayed until it took effect. Attempts to explain what was happening to Mrs Jones were unsuccessful because of her dementia and she became very agitated. As a result she flailed as the doctor was injecting the local anaesthetic, causing her arm to bleed. Despite the anaesthetic and analgesic, it was clear that Mrs Jones was in a considerable amount of pain when her wrist was manipulated. She wriggled a lot and started shouting. At this point the doctor, who was holding Mrs Jones' left hand, asked me to hold her left arm above the elbow to keep her still enough for the cast to be applied.

This incident provoked a number of feelings in me. Firstly, I was confused about the lack of communication regarding the procedure – the nursing team had been under the impression that a general anaesthetic was to be used. During the procedure I felt useless; there was little I could do to assist apart from helping to hold Mrs Jones still and attempting to reassure and distract her. Most of all I felt guilty because as a team we were causing the patient so much pain. I felt worse knowing that it wasn't just the orthopaedic procedure that was causing her pain but also our attempts to keep her still. I also felt slightly angry because, as a student ODP on observation, I did not feel able to question the events in any way.

On the positive side, Mrs Jones was asleep half an hour after the procedure, remembered nothing of the event and returned to her nursing home the next day. I gained empirical knowledge, observed an orthopaedic procedure done under local that I would not have seen otherwise and learned a little about the realities of dealing with patients with dementia. Usually when these patients come to theatre they are heavily sedated and we don't have to cope with their behaviour, even in the recovery room. On the negative side, though, the incident could have been handled a lot better. Firstly, the lack of communication resulted in Mrs Jones being nil-by-mouth for 13 hours. Not only was this unnecessary and must have caused discomfort, it could also result in dehydration, which interferes with normal bodily processes. Where a patient is unable to communicate effectively with the caring staff this is even more dangerous and could have serious consequences. Secondly, it resulted in inadequate sedation and analgesia, causing Mrs Jones more pain and distress than she should have had.

*Case study continued*

I have learned a great deal from this incident in terms of the need to treat patients individually. This often gets overlooked in theatres as patients are listed for procedures and we rarely interact with them as people. Reducing this fracture under general anaesthetic would have been an easier and more straightforward procedure but was not the most appropriate course of action for Mrs Jones because of her age and anaesthetic risk. My role under these circumstances was different from my normal one, and yet it is becoming more likely given the expanding role of ODPs into different clinical situations. I have realised that I take comfort from the fact that patients are usually unconscious and that I don't have to offer emotional support or think about not causing them pain. I appreciate now the role that nurses often play in reassuring and supporting patients in order to reduce anxiety and gain co-operation, and that these are skills that I will need to learn. This placement has been a very valuable learning experience in that I now see people more as individuals with different needs than simply as procedures on a list.

All clinical placements will offer you alternative experiences and will have been chosen, and audited, for their potential educational value in contributing to your experience. Sometimes you may be disappointed that you have not got the placement that you wanted, but making the most of what the placement offers is an important skill to develop, despite your feelings about it. Planning to use the placement for what it can offer you and how it can help you to achieve your learning outcomes is a positive way of approaching new placements. We can do this by analysing the context of the placement and anticipating the types of opportunities and experiences that it can offer. The following checklist will help you in doing this.

---

### Check list to use in evaluating the potential of a clinical placement

- What is the specialty of the placement?
- What are the characteristics of the patients it deals with in terms of:
  - age
  - sex
  - reason for being a patient and/or
  - reason for being under the care of your professional group
  - other specific criteria, e.g. immobility, disability?
- What is the range of experience that it can offer you?
- What specific experiences and/or events are available here?
- What skills/competencies will you achieve here?
- How will this placement contribute to your overall course outcomes?

Much of your learning in placements will come from specific events, such as critical incidents, that happen to you.

**Key points** Top tips

- Placements are unique and offer unique experiences
- Analyse your placements to identify what they can offer against your learning needs
- Plan to use your placements to achieve your objectives

## Learning from events

Clearly, whenever you are in placements in the clinical environment, things will be going on around you all the time. In fact, so much will be happening that you will find it impossible to take everything in that happens while you are there! There are two ways that we can look at this.

Firstly, we can allow things to wash over us and just experience them as they happen. This is what we will do most of the time, and we will slowly absorb the ways of working and doing things as we become familiar with what is going on.

Secondly, however, we may consciously decide to focus on events that are happening and make them a feature of our reflective practice. In these instances we will be selecting from everything that is happening for a particular purpose.

In the second case, the reasons we decide to concentrate on a particular event are important. Some of these reasons may be:

- It is selected for you by your supervisor because it is something that they feel you need to do at that time
- Because you need to experience and learn one thing before you are able to go on and do others
- Because that event happens irregularly and therefore you need to make the most of when it does occur
- Because different skills or ways of doing something will be on offer that your supervisor feels will broaden your experience
- Because you have specific learning outcomes for that placement
- Because this experience is only likely to be available from this placement.

Making the most of events that are occurring is important in enabling you to get the most from what is on offer. Many experiences cannot be predicted; others can. It is up to you, along with your supervisor, to ensure that you select from what is available in any placement to ensure that you gain the experiences that you need as a practitioner. One of the ways in which you may identify these is through your course competencies and the outcomes expected for professional registration.

---

**Key points**  *Top tips*

- Analyse each placement for the specific events that occur that you need or want to experience
- Arrange your placement time/shifts so that you are there when they happen
- Tell your supervisor, or the other people that you are working with, if there is anything that you want to be able to experience while on that placement

---

## Learning from course structure, competencies and course outcomes

Your course will be organised and structured in a way to ensure that you experience and achieve what you need in order to qualify in your chosen profession. How this is structured derives from the experience of your lecturers and supervisors in practice. Similarly, the placements that are organised for you will have been done so with specific objectives in mind. After all, you cannot learn everything at once! Each unit, or module of study, will have specified learning outcomes. Similarly, your stage in the course provides expectations about your knowledge, skills and what you can do in the practical environment. You will be expected to build on foundational skills and knowledge as you progress through the course, incrementally developing your way to competence as a practitioner in your own right.

Using outcomes to structure your learning experiences is a useful way of ensuring that you achieve everything that you need. By identifying what it is that you need to achieve, you can assess what is on offer in a particular placement and plan to achieve the outcomes, or competencies, that will be available there. This does take active planning and review at specific points during the placement to assess whether you are on track. Both your clinical supervisor and academic tutor will be available to help you with this.

With all of these having been given to you, your main job is to make the most of the opportunities that are presented to you in the clinical environment. This will ensure that you learn from the broadest possible range of experiences that are available in your protected time as a pre-qualifying student. This will happen if you spend some of your private study time planning what it is that you need to achieve, and how you will do this during the different stages of your course.

> ### Over to you
>
> Construct a checklist for evaluating specific events that you may come across in your placements. Use the one in the previous section to provide cue questions that you can use when selecting and reflecting on events that may be available as experiences in placements. Try to relate these to your course or module outcomes; to assignments that you may need to complete; or to clinical or practical competencies.

It may be that you can use one event for several different purposes. For instance, reflecting on one critical incident may enable you to provide evidence of having achieved a couple of competencies, and satisfy a written course work assignment demonstrating your ability to use a reflective framework. This whole piece of work may then be included in your portfolio as evidence of your ongoing development and gradual achievement of the course outcomes. Using the same event for different outcomes also enables you to see the links between theory and practice, and the integration of the different components of the course. Reflective processes and practice are not strategies that can be separated out from the reality of being a practitioner. They cannot occur in the abstract because they depend on real life for their subject matter. So, although you are being encouraged to focus specifically on them while a student, they are like any other skill or technique that you use in your professional development in that they do not stand alone but, rather, are incorporated into everything you do.

### Key points | Top tips

- Use the information that you have been given about your course structure, assignments and competencies to plan to get the most out of your clinical placements
- Spend time at the beginning of the placement in planning what you will be able to achieve from what you need to achieve

## Self-directed learning and individual interests

Finally, your own interests and needs will help to provide some direction in selecting what you choose to use as active learning experiences. These might arise from your evaluation of what your strengths and weaknesses are, of where your own professional interests lie or of the type of specialty that you want to go into when you qualify. The time you spend on your course will provide you with a range of opportunities that you are unlikely to encounter in such a short space of time again in your career. While the purpose of your course is to enable you to develop an acceptable level of competence as a practitioner so that you can safely be allowed to be responsible for patient care, your registration as a practitioner is simply the beginning of another stage in your learning.

After qualification you will begin to build your skills, knowledge and expertise directed by your own interests and aptitudes, as opposed to those directed for you by the needs of registration and regulation. This flexibility brings with it another set of responsibilities as you become your own guide for your professional learning needs. This process starts, like all others, during the pre-qualifying period, in that there will always be self-identified and self-directed learning needs that arise over and above those specified in your course. It is likely that many of these will arise from the experiences that you have in clinical placements. As you find that you want to know more about what you are encountering, you will realise that the generic knowledge learned in college is insufficient for the specific experiences that occur in the real world of patient care. Thus, much of your reflective learning from clinical placements will arise from the unique experiences that you have throughout your course. Using these as a focus for reflective practice will therefore broaden your base for professional practice.

Your self-directed and independent learning, just like all the other opportunities that you have, will need to be focused in particular ways. As a student, this is usually done by screening out things that are not essential to success in your course. Hence, when selecting what to spend your self-directed time on, you will need to ask yourself specific, needs-related questions and be quite instrumental in how you use your time. You will find that you can 'double-count' much of what you are doing by ensuring that you use many, if not all, of what you do for at least two purposes. Many of these incidences will arise by combining the requirements of your course with your own interests. You might, for instance:

- Choose to focus an assignment on a subject matter that is of specific interest to you
- Select a critical incident that enables you to explore your own interests while achieving several competencies or learning outcomes in the course
- Ensure that the topic of your final project or dissertation is related to the specialty of the placement/s you will be in at the time
- Select elective placements, particularly towards the end of your course, that enable you to develop skills and contacts for employment on qualification.

---

### Over to you

We all have criteria that help us decide how we will use our time. Try to develop a list of your own that will guide your self-directed study and that reflects your needs as a student in planning to complete your course successfully. The following questions may help you to do this, but you will probably want to add more of your own.

- Why have I chosen to read/study/write about this topic?
- How does it fit with the stage/requirements of the course at this moment?
- How will it help me to achieve this semester's/year's academic assignments?
- How will it inform my practical placements?
- How will it contribute to my knowledge for my future practice?
- Does it contribute to the competencies I need to demonstrate?
- What am I trying to achieve in doing it?
- Do I have the time to do it?
- Do I really need to do it?
- Do I really want to do it?

---

As you progress through your course, you will find that you are drawn to some elements of practice more than others and that these are where you choose to specialise when you qualify. The nature of most professional practice in contemporary health care means that practitioners choose specialist areas of practice very soon after qualification. For many of you this will not be a conscious decision. This may be because you have a broad range of interests and do not have any particular leanings towards one or another. Others know at an early stage in their course just where their interests lie and choose to specialise swiftly after initial qualification by going on to further courses or working in designated areas of their practice. These areas of interest are often founded in our pre-qualifying experiences.

---

**Key points** ~~Top tips~~

- We learn best where our interest is stimulated – so try to focus as much of your required course components as you can though your own specific interests
- We tend to be 'needs' motivated as students – in other words, we focus our time on to what we need to do, rather than what we want to do. If we can find ways of combining these, and double counting our experiences in clinical environments, we are more likely to achieve our goals successfully
- Your pre-qualifying course is simply a preparation for the rest of your professional life – so try to use your clinical experiences constructively for the future. Look out for opportunities that will establish the foundations for your career as a practitioner

---

## Conclusions

The learning achieved from your clinical experiences and placements is the link between theory and practice. As practitioners we can only make sense of theory if we apply it, see it in action, reflect on it and discover our own knowledge base derived from this unique combination. Every practitioner has a different knowledge base for practice arising from the experiences they have had – no two practitioners have ever had the same experiential basis for their learning. Hence, no two practitioners can be said to have the same knowledge base. As practitioners, our skill lies in safe and competent practice, in being able to select from alternatives and predict outcomes for our patients. We need to have confidence in and justify our professional decisions and actions. We need to acknowledge the limitations of our own practice and be prepared to listen to others, or invite them in to share the care of our patients. None of this can be learned from theory alone.

As a student you have the privilege of being able to study in the real world. Within this world there is a wealth of opportunities available for learning your craft. These range from the people you meet, to the specialist services encountered, the events and experiences that happen opportunistically or as planned occurrences, and our natural tendencies in terms of interests and motivation.

The key to getting the most out of clinical placements and environments is in planning your experiences to ensure that you identify the opportunities they offer and maximising how they help you to achieve your outcomes. Reflective processes and practice provide the strategies for you to do this, whether these are used in anticipation of your clinical experiences or retrospectively after events have occurred.

---

## ʀʀʀʀʀ*Rapid recap*

Check your progress so far by working through each of the following questions.
1. What is the primary difference between the college environment and the practice environment?
2. To whom do you have responsibilities in the clinical environment?
3. What are your roles as a student in the practice environment?
4. What is meant by 'self-empowerment'?
5. What are the different types of learning opportunities available in clinical practice?
6. What is meant by the term 'socialisation processes'?
7. How can we get the most out of the opportunities available for learning in practice?

If you have difficulty with more than one of the questions, read through the section again to refresh your understanding before moving on.

# Ways of reflecting on your own

While the previous chapters have worked at setting up the foundations for and ideas behind reflective practice, these next two present practical ways of actually being a reflective practitioner.

The aim of this chapter is to introduce you to a variety of strategies for reflecting by yourself. We start by revisiting the idea of actively working with your learning style, before moving on to the two principal ways in which you will reflect by yourself – thinking things over and writing reflectively. While both these approaches share common elements, they each have individual features that contribute separately to the techniques you will use to learn and understand about practice. Some use the frameworks for reflection introduced in Chapter 3; others are more creative and therefore provide a range of approaches for the different situations in which you find yourself reflecting, and for the differing purposes for reflecting in the first place. It is important for you to build up a 'kit-bag' of reflective strategies, some formal, others less so, as ways of learning from your practice and experiences throughout your course. One strategy is not necessarily appropriate for all situations. As a result, this chapter and the next explore the very practical aspects of reflecting, enabling you to select from different approaches depending on the context in which you are reflecting and what you want to achieve from it.

Most reflection will be done on your own. At the end of the day, reflection is a solitary learning activity and, while other people can help you to do it, the insights and learning that will be achieved will be just yours. The ways in which you achieve these, however, can be many and varied. At the outset of your reflective journey it is worth remembering that, just as there are many routes and means of transport to get yourself from A to B, there are also many strategies that you can use for reflection.

## Working with your learning style

In Chapter 2 you worked through the activity of identifying your learning style. We ended that section by presenting a table of the learning activities that suit each particular style (Table 2.5, p. 57). We want to return to this briefly, so that you can begin to think about the types of reflective strategy that will most suit your style, and actively work to develop these. A word of caution, though – as with all diagnostic and labelling tools, this one is only meant to give you an insight, and some ideas about how you can use the tendencies identified. Just because you appear to 'fit' mostly into one preferred learning style or another does not mean that you need to try to alter who and what you are. Nor does it mean that you necessarily operate from that basis at all times, as clearly everyone is a mixture of all the features. Your preferred learning style, therefore, is where most of your tendencies lie, based on the answers you gave on the day that you completed the questions. This does not mean that you are fixed in this, nor that you cannot work to move consciously from one style to another.

### *Reflective activity*

You've now had some time between identifying your learning style in Chapter 2 and working with it through Chapters 3 and 4. So perhaps it's a good time to reflect back on your reactions to doing that activity and what you might have discovered about yourself.

Firstly, did the preferred learning style category that you fell into provide any shocks? Did you have a mental picture of the category that you would have liked to have been in? Were these the same? If not, has falling into a different category made you think at all about:

- Your perception of yourself
- The ways in which you go about your learning?

Secondly, look back at Table 2.5 on p. 57 and consider the types of activity suggested for your learning style. How many of these would you consciously say were 'you'? How many did you read and think 'No, I wouldn't want to do that'?

Now scan the activities suggested for the other learning styles. How many of these appeal to you as well?

You should now have a list of the types of activity that you can plan to use that will suit your learning style, and therefore engage your interest and motivation. All of these can be used actively within reflective practice, so keep this list at hand and plan to incorporate some of these activities in the way that you reflect when by yourself.

- Being aware of your learning style enables you to select the methods for learning through reflection that will suit you most
- Planning your reflective learning through different kinds of activity will maintain your interest and maximise your learning from your experiences

## Thinking things over

Much of the reflection that you do will be inside your head. It is here that the distinction between reflection-in-action and reflection-on-action will become most apparent.

### Reflection-in-action

It is clear that we cannot be aware of our thought and decision-making processes every time we do something – at the very least we wouldn't get anything done! But, there are times when we are aware of consciously thinking about alternatives to action and actively selecting from them while we are doing it. For instance, you may be having a conversation with a patient but at the same time be thinking 'What's going on here?', 'What might be the reason for this?' or 'What is the best way of dealing with this?'

When you start in your practice placements, you will probably be more aware of reflecting-in-action because the situations will be unfamiliar. As a result of this you will have to work hard at understanding what is going on and have to think through many of your actions before you do them. Take, for instance, what Kim says in the following case study.

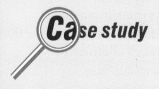

**Case study**

### Kim's experience

I was going to take Mrs G's blood pressure. While placing the cuff around her upper arm I noticed that there was little length on the cuff to accommodate its circumference. Knowing there was a larger cuff on another trolley, I glanced down the ward to see if it was free, but it was in use, so I made the decision to continue with the one I had. When I inflated the cuff the Velcro fastening began to rip and eventually the cuff came flying off. Mrs G looked at me and made a comment about having 'fat arms'. I made light of the situation, apologised and waited for the larger cuff.

This is a simple example of reflecting-in-action. Unfortunately, Kim made an inappropriate decision, even though she had thought things through in the first place. Her decision-making was flawed as she was not thinking in the best interests of the patient or in clinical terms about obtaining the most accurate reading, but in terms of inconvenience.

You will often find yourself reflecting-in-action, and it is worth making a mental note of those occasions so that you are aware that you are practising reflectively. You may also like to take note of when you tend to practise in a routine way, or do things because you are told to do them. It is very easy, especially as a beginning practitioner, to allow feelings of insecurity and wanting to fit in to influence the actions you take, rather than actually stopping to think about whether these are the best courses of action to take. A cue for you to stop and think is when you feel uncomfortable about doing what others have asked you to do, or when you are aware that things are being done in a way that is incorrect. For instance, Ann was helping a staff nurse with a procedure.

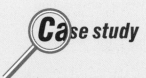

### Ann's experience

She was going to pass the nasogastric tube, but I realised that she didn't have gloves on. We had been taught that for both patients' and our own protection, any procedures like this should be done with gloves. I suppose she had just got into the habit of not doing some things with gloves. Also, there is often a shortage of gloves, so the nurses are careful about when they use them. Anyway, I pointed this out, and asked whether there was a reason for her decision, as I didn't want her to feel I was picking her up. She replied that she had actually forgotten them and thanked me for reminding her.

Reflecting-in-action in this way contributes to 'thoughtful' practice, or the ways that responsible practitioners think in action. It is what, to some extent, identifies professional practitioners from unqualified staff, as they are constantly sifting through alternatives in their head to determine the best and most appropriate care. Most reflecting-in-action is done unconsciously, or without us being aware of it. It becomes the way that practitioners practise automatically (Rolfe *et al.* 2001). But initially, by being aware of doing this, you will not only be taking steps to becoming a professional practitioner but you are more likely to make the most appropriate decisions for your patients.

> ### Over to you
>
> Next time you are in practice, talk to your supervisor, or any other person you are working with, about the way that they use reflection-in-action. You may find that you need to explain what you are talking about first, as many practitioners may not be aware of the theoretical concept of reflection-in-action. However, once you explain, it is more than likely that they will know exactly what you are talking about and can give you plenty of examples of the ways in which they use reflection-in-action throughout their working day.

Reflecting-in-action helps to safeguard against routinised practice and leads us towards conscious awareness of our actions and decisions in practice. It is the way in which we can deliver individualised, rather than generalised, care that is tailored to the unique needs of each patient. What it can also do is provide us with the material for reflecting-on-action.

## Reflection-on-action

Reflection-on-action is the process that we are more likely to be aware of when we are reflecting. It occurs after the event, rather than as it is happening (see Chapter 1 for a definition). Reflection-on-action is the main way that you will be using reflective practice overtly throughout your course, as you reflect by yourself, with and for others.

Reflecting-on-action as a thoughtful activity may happen quite spontaneously, or be something that you take time to do deliberately. Either way, there is a difference between using the reflective cycle to explore experiences and simply thinking them over in your head.

When we use reflective practice, we are reflecting for two main purposes:

- To learn from the experience
- To frame action that we will take.

These two features differentiate active reflection-on-action from the mulling over that goes on in our heads most of the time, which is mistakenly considered by many practitioners to be reflective practice. You may hear other people say that they 'do' reflective practice all the time, but what they really mean is that they think about what they are doing. Reflective practice as a conscious activity is a great deal more than that, as you will have already come to realise.

Deliberate reflection-on-action helps us to develop our understanding of situations so that we can learn from them and change our practice for the future. When we create time to do this we are choosing to use our time to make sense of our experiences.

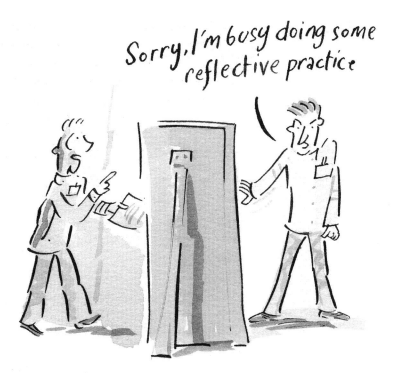

*There is more to true and effective reflective practice than you might think*

Time is a valuable resource for most of us, and therefore deserves to be put to good use. So, when you do set aside time to reflect, it is worth ensuring that you plan to use it effectively and for some purpose.

Most of the activities that you have met so far in this book have asked you to engage in some sort of reflection by using cue questions. The purpose of this was to start you reflecting without the mystique and aura of it being 'reflective practice'. Hopefully, by now you will have realised that there are many different ways of reflecting, and not all of them are confined to structures and strategies. You can learn just as much from purposefully thinking issues through, provided you identify the learning and take some action as a result. However, you can also learn by working through a framework for reflection, and when you start out in reflective practice this might be a way of organising both the reflective processes and your thoughts. Once you understand what it is that you are trying to achieve, and plan to use the reflective mechanisms to do this, it will become second nature.

So, how do we do it? This is more difficult to help you with, for the simple reason that, if we provide you with examples, it becomes written reflection, which is dealt with in the next section! What we can do, though, is to show you how others use contemplative reflection-on-action to make sense of their experiences, and hope that this will provide you with clues as to how you can use it yourself. The other way is to go back to your preferred learning style and ask yourself how you can incorporate reflection-on-action within that.

## Case study

### Kim's experience (continued)

Do you remember Kim's experience when taking Mrs G's blood pressure? As well as reflecting-in-action, she made a point of thinking things through more deeply later on. The reasons she did this were that:

● She was embarrassed that she had caused Mrs G distress

● She realised that the procedure had not been effective

● She realised that she had made the wrong decision in choosing to carry on using the standard cuff.

● As she said:

*At the time I was thinking that the procedure would not be successful and I should stop using the cuff, but then part of me argued that there was maybe a chance that it would work and to wait for the outcome. I also knew we were under pressure to get the obs done, and were short-staffed, and waiting for the other cuff would delay things.*

Kim used Johns's structured model of reflection to think her way through the incident and rationalise what she had done. She came to further understandings about it, and managed to see clearly where her priorities had been at that time. She was very concerned about the distress and embarrassment that she had caused Mrs G, especially as it was in front of the other patients. She realised that it was this concern that prompted her to think about the way she delivered care, and that perhaps she had fallen into the trap of practising routinely rather than really thinking about what she was doing with each patient.

**Her learning:** Kim realised that the delivery of individualised care has to be a deliberate and considered activity, otherwise care is routine. She learned that sometimes she does not put the patient at the front of her care decisions and delivery.

**Her action:** She resolved to never make decisions based on time and inconvenience again. She vowed that she would try to look at patients' individual needs when delivering care.

This process took Kim about 5 minutes, as she was able to sit quietly during her coffee break after the incident and reflect on what had happened. Despite the fact that it took so little time, the understanding that Kim developed, and her resolve to change her actions, will have long-lasting consequences for her future practice.

Reflective activity of this sort need not take a lot of time, and a lack of time is no excuse for not thinking incidents and experiences over reflectively after they have occurred. It is not as though you will need to reflect in this way on everything that happens to you. But making reflection-on-action a habitual part of your practice will help you in developing your own knowledge and understanding for your practice. At the end of the day, it will probably actually save you time, because the learning achieved and the changes you make to your practice are immediate.

---

### Over to you

Reflection-on-action in this way has to be a deliberate activity. You have to take the decision to do it – no-one can force you. So, it really is over to you this time! Will you rise to the challenge of trying to reflect on at least one incident or experience every day you are in practice?

---

### Key points Top tips

- Reflection-in-action occurs as we are working, and is often unconscious
- By deliberating taking notice of when we are using reflection-in-action we will be aware of and maximise our learning
- Reflection-in-action can be seen as 'thoughtful practice'
- Reflection-on-action is a deliberate activity that occurs after the event
- We need to make time to use reflection-on-action by ourselves as thinking things over
- Getting into the habit of mentally reviewing and reflecting on experiences every day will begin the process of developing reflective practice
- Reflection-on-action is more than simply thinking about our practice
- Reflective practice is about identifying our learning and taking action as a result of using the ERA cycle

○━┳ *Keywords*

**Reflective writing**
Writing for the purpose of
learning from experience

# Reflective writing

The other way we can use the reflective processes within our learning
is through writing reflectively. This has a different character and
process from thinking things through reflectively and, although it
is probably less prevalent in professional practice on a day-to-day
basis, it is an extremely valuable way of learning from practice and
becoming a consciously reflective practitioner. It is also the way that
you will provide evidence to others of your development.

## Writing reflectively

As a student, you will be required to record much of your reflective
activity. This may take various forms and formats, and these will often
be provided for you, such as in reflective reviews, portfolio entries or
essay formats exploring a particular incident or element of practice.
So far you have met many different strategies and approaches to
reflection in this book, from structured reflection through various
different models to reflection that you may choose from as a strategy
for learning and uncovering knowledge. In this section we explore the
value of written reflection, or deliberately using strategies of writing as
a way of reflecting and as a way of learning from experience. This is,
of course, used with any of the frameworks identified in Chapter 3,
which will provide you with structures through which you can order
your thoughts and writing. Writing can be used to 'add value' to the
reflective work that you may do in your head, or with others.

## What is *reflective* writing?

Reflective writing involves engaging in, and completing, the reflective
cycle using writing processes to help you learn. **Reflective writing**
differs from other forms of writing only in that it has one primary
purpose – that of learning – to enable you to come to a different, or
deeper, understanding of whatever you are reflecting on. The other
results of writing, such as having a record of what you have done,
or completing an assignment, are supplementary to this, and it is
worth bearing this in mind when creating strategies for reflective
writing for yourself – or, indeed, doing the writing itself.

**Keywords**

**Transformative**
Changing or developing the
ways in which we see things

## Reflective activity

### The last time you wrote

Think back to the last time you wrote a piece of academic work.
Draw a line down the middle of your page. On the left hand side try to
answer the following questions about what you wrote.

1. What did you write?

2. What was the purpose (why did you write it)?

3. How did you decide what, and what not, to write?

4. How did you decide on the order of what you wrote?

5. How did you organise or structure what you wrote?

On the right hand side of the page try to think about the 'why' questions – why
were you writing, why did you include some things and leave others out? Why did
you order it in this way? Why did you organise what you were writing in this way?

Now, try to think a bit deeper about the process of writing itself and what was
going on while you were writing. Did the act of writing as a mental activity enable
other things to happen? For instance, if you were writing an essay, did you find
that you were drawing conclusions that you didn't realise you had reached? If
you were writing a reflective review, did you remember things in the descriptive
stage that you had previously forgotten? If you were writing a report on a client,
did you start to make connections between things that you hadn't seen before?

Finally, what, for you, makes the process of writing different from the
processes used in thinking things over in your head?

We asked you to think about what happened as a result of the
process of your writing – whether you added something to your
work that wasn't previously there, or whether you began to see
something in a different light as a result of writing. This provides an
illustration of the **transformative** nature of writing when viewed
from the *writing-to-learn* perspective (Allen *et al.* 1989) – the act of
writing in itself adds to the way in which we view our experiences.
We can actively plan to use this feature of writing when we choose
to write reflectively.

## Features of reflective writing

Reflective writing can be seen as building on and developing the skills
that we already have in other forms of writing. When using reflective
writing, we might think about the following features.

### The reason we are writing

We always write for some purpose, even if it is simply a note
reminding someone to get the washing in if it rains. Not only is writing
purposeful, it is also deliberate – we have to decide to write, and give

all of our attention to it at the time, as few thoughts, other than very simple things such as 'Do I need another cup of coffee?' can be going on in our heads at the same time. This combination of thinking, and translating those thoughts into writing, involves complex mental and physical processes that force us to focus completely on what we are doing. When we decide to write reflectively, we need to create the time and space to do so, as with any other type of writing; in other words, we make a commitment of our time and energy to the writing. Writing reflectively is a deliberate strategy to commit ourselves to identifying our learning, and framing action as a result. The consequences of this are that when we write we make a commitment to both the content and process of what we are writing. When writing reflectively this commitment becomes all important, in that we need a stimulus or a purpose for doing it and very often this arises from within ourselves and our practice.

### How we can use writing to help order our thoughts

Secondly, writing forces us to impose some sort of order on the content of what we are writing. The order for some reflective writing will be given to you, by the lecturers you are writing for as part of your course, by a reflective model or perhaps by a portfolio structure. For less formal writing, however, you have the freedom to write in whatever way you want, because the writing only needs to make sense to yourself.

The process of writing helps us to find both a structure for its content and an order for the points we want to make. Therefore, it also helps us to prioritise and identify what is important and what is not within the writing. How does this work? One reason is that our writing speed is limited by our typing speed or how fast we can physically write. This is slower than the speed at which we think, therefore we are slowed down in our thinking as we mentally sift and segregate the most important things to write. We cannot write at the speed we think, or even at the speed we talk; thus writing reflectively will be very different in content and structure from the way we reflect when talking to others or by ourselves contemplatively. It has three distinct features that can be seen as an advantage:

- We are forced to acknowledge issues that may be ignored if we are carrying on a conversation or reflecting inside our heads
- We can put a hierarchical order to issues that are significant to us
- This enables us to work through these issues as we have identified them, rather than being side-tracked into other things.

These make reflective writing an extremely personal process, and one that helps us to work systematically through a process of reflection.

This differs from simply thinking things through, where we may get stuck going round and round in circles in our head.

### The purpose of creating a permanent record

Although this point may seem obvious, writing creates a permanent record that can be returned to and reconsidered. It is important because:

- **It helps to provide a fuller picture of what has gone on.** The act of writing helps us to remember not only things we think we have forgotten but also things that may be hidden or overlaid by others that take priority. In trying to recall things that have happened to us and recount them verbally we are selective in what we remember – the problem of hindsight bias. Very often we are convinced that we have remembered every detail, yet others who were also there at the time might say 'Yes, but do you remember this too…'. Thus writing will jog our memory and fill in another piece of the jigsaw puzzle.

- **In writing things down we record what our memory allows us to remember at the time.** This might be close to the event, or at some time distant. This creates at least one account of the event, which can be used in the future for reflective activity. This original description can act as a memory jogger the next time you read it, when more, or different details and explanations of what has happened occur to us.

- **The written record allows us to put the event away and return to it at a later date.** As a result of the time and space created we are often able to take a different perspective on the event and see it in a different way, by filling in more information or considering it in the light of new or alternative experiences and knowledge.

- **In writing things down we cannot ignore or forget them.** Rolfe *et al.* provide the anecdote of one student who said that:

  *an advantage in writing things down was that it made you deal with them, unlike being able to ignore them if they are in your head. He said that once they had appeared on paper there was a constant reminder and this acted as a prompt to sort them out, and that to some extent this was a hidden effect of writing – that it acted as a conscience so that you couldn't conveniently forget things – that they may turn out to be the key to a problem that you haven't yet found.*

  Rolfe *et al.* 2001, p. 51

### How we can be creative through writing

Writing in itself can be creative. How often have you sat down with the intention of writing one thing and ended up with something completely different? This is why many academic tutors suggest that the introduction to a piece of written work is the last part to be written – so that you can ensure that you introduce the work that is presented, and not the work you intended to write! Our mind takes us down paths as a result of considering the material in front of us at that particular time – it helps us to create an alternative, and sometimes unexpected, sense of what we are seeing. Thus we may make connections between pieces of information that in the past we had not contemplated. The writing process helps us to *integrate* disparate information sets into new combinations, enabling us to take a different perspective on an issue. Writing may lead to creative thinking, where not only can you justify and defend your actions, but you may also develop new understandings and perspectives on a situation, or come to understand a past event in a different light.

### Using writing to develop our analytical skills

One of the effects of increasing the amount of writing that we do is that we get more used to being analytical in how we do it. It really is one of those things that gets easier the more you do! Initially when you start writing reflectively you will probably find that you want the structure provided for you by some sort of a reflective framework. However, as you get used to ordering the different elements in your head, and reviewing your experiences through the reflective processes, you will find that you start to experiment with the frameworks or decide to omit some stages as you go along. You may find that you adapt a framework to make it 'fit' more closely with the type of experience you are reflecting on, or the purpose that you want to fulfil. You may even end up creating your own framework, especially if you move beyond the confines of using only critical incidents that have happened, into using reflective practice in a predictive way.

When we analyse, we break things down into their component parts. We learn to see those components as separate elements and consider their role in relation to the whole. Some parts will be more important, or significant, for what we are learning than others. The features of writing that we have already identified, for creating a permanent record and providing an order to our thoughts, also aid us in becoming more analytical. They do this by giving us the means to break things down through a framework or specific structure that the experience itself did not possess. We record the experience descriptively, as we perceived it. We then analyse our description by identifying and building on the separate features of it. The written record provides us with a way of slowing this process down, as our

**o—ᴙ *Keywords***

**Critical thinking**
The processes involved in
exploring and weighing up
possibilities for action and
making a rational choice

fingers try to keep up with our brain. This, in turn, makes us stop and think differently, or more deeply. This is in contrast to when we sit and think things through without writing, as there are no mental stops where we say 'What am I going to write next?' or 'What did that really mean?' or 'Did I really say that?'

**Using writing to develop our critical thinking**

Within the reflective cycle, being critical about our experiences follows on from the analytical stages. By this we do not mean finding fault or being negative, but taking an objective stance to exploring something in a balanced way. Many writers see the reflective process as key to developing **critical thinking**, and reflective writing as a crucial process of enabling it to happen. Critical thinking is also regarded as crucial to the ways in which practitioners make decisions about their practice.

Critical thinking has been defined as: 'The process of purposeful, self-regulatory judgement; an interactive reflective, reasoning process' (Facione *et al*. 1994, p. 345). It is a complicated, complex and intricate process that involves problem-solving, reasoning in considering opposing viewpoints or competing theories and an attitude of inquiry.

So, critical thinking is about weighing up all the possibilities for action and being able to make a reasoned and rational choice. Brookfield (1987) has identified the features of people who are critical thinkers as:

- Engaging in productive and positive activity
- Viewing their thinking as a process rather than an outcome
- Varying in their manifestations of critical thinking according to context
- Experiencing triggers to critical thinking as positive or negative
- Feeling comfortable with the emotive as well as the rational elements of the critical thinking process.

So how can reflective writing help us to become critical thinkers? If we think back to the processes of the reflective cycle, we can see that in choosing to adopt these we will automatically be working in the ways that critical thinkers work. Brookfield (1987) defines the components of critical thinking as:

- **Identifying and challenging assumptions:** This means ensuring that you write down the assumptions that you made in relation to an event that you describe. These assumptions may be the knowledge or theory that you used, or particular paradigm cases that you can remember, or experiential learning.

- **Recognising the importance of context:** Our actions are never context-free – we all work within the confines of our experiences of the world, time and place that we have lived. These ultimately interfere with and affect the way in which we see others. Exploring the context of events and acknowledging the limitations of our perceptions enables us to think more analytically, and therefore critically. Writing these down provides us with a way of objectifying our experiences; we are able to stand outside the experiences as personal and view them from a different perspective.

- **Exploring and imagining alternatives:** Critical thinking involves being able to compare and evaluate different solutions to problems, or consider events in order to uncover new and different ways of perceiving the world. Writing enables us to explore and imagine alternative viewpoints by providing us with structures and questions which challenge our previous way of looking at things.

- **Reflective scepticism:** Being sceptical protects us from accepting 'universal truths' or that there is only ever one explanation for an event or one way of looking at it. Developing scepticism leads us to question and seek alternative answers – it may lead ultimately to the development of new understandings by encouraging us to reject previously accepted explanations.

Each of these is incorporated within the reflective cycle; hence, in choosing to write reflectively, we will also be developing our powers of critical thinking.

### Using writing to develop new understandings and knowledge

The processes of writing can help us to develop our understanding of what we are experiencing, and may lead us to create new knowledge for ourselves. This can happen at any stage of the reflective cycle because the very process of ordering the way we write things down may create a new way of seeing things or provide a new perspective.

### Using writing to show that we understand something

We cannot write convincingly about things that we do not understand. By being able to write about them we show ourselves that we can explain it and understand it. How often have you tried to explain something to someone else, and at the end realised that you knew more than you thought you did? Or conversely, how often have you found yourself rambling through an explanation for something and ending up confusing your listener even more because you hadn't really got the important points straight in your head? Writing also has this effect. If you can write a clear description and analysis of the experience you are reflecting on, it will provide you with more clarity about it. You will cut out all the extraneous information and focus, in the end, on the key elements for your learning and action for practice.

### Writing in the first person

If we are writing about things that have happened to us personally, or in relation to ourselves, it is obvious that we need to write in the first person. This means writing using 'I'. This makes us take responsibility for our part in the experience, and acknowledge our role in what has happened. It also helps to avoid blaming other people for what happened, because their part will be located in the descriptive part of the account. The purpose of reflective writing is personal (usually); therefore, it is our own behaviour that needs to be the focus of the writing. It is clearly nonsense to try to write reflectively in the third person, or to take yourself out of your account. Equally, it is unreasonable to try to change the behaviour of others, so try to avoid saying 'They should have …'; clearly, they didn't, and it isn't your concern, other than as a point of learning.

---

## Reflective activity

Take some time to think about what you have just read about the nature of reflective writing and how it is different from thinking things through.

How does this, as a reflective strategy, interlink with your preferred learning style?

Can you identify an example from your practice that you would choose to consider using written reflection rather than thoughtful reflection? What might be the advantages of one method of reflection over the other?

---

The features of writing are significant for how we learn. But writing reflectively involves more than simply 'writing things down': it often involves the analysis and identification of the roles we have played in events in our lives. But this depends on what we are reflecting on and the purpose we want the reflection to achieve. Just as reflective writing as a whole can be used in different ways by people with different learning styles, it is important to remember that no one strategy will suit everyone. Equally, there is no right and wrong about reflective writing and the adoption of a technique that is contrary to your own personality, learning style and inclination is likely to be doomed to failure from the start. In the next section we present a selection of ways that you can use to write reflectively.

- Reflective writing is writing that is done for the purpose of learning
- Reflective writing builds on the unique features of writing in creating artefacts that can be used
- Reflective writing can be used within any of the preferred learning styles

## Styles and strategies for reflective writing

Rolfe *et al.* (2001) provide a basic framework that divides strategies for reflective writing into two basic types – analytical strategies and creative strategies. These are summarised in Table 5.1.

| Table 5.1 **Strategies for reflective writing (adapted from Rolfe *et al.* 2001)** | |
| --- | --- |
| **Analytical strategies** | **Creative strategies** |
| Learning journals | Writing the unsent letter, memo or e-mail |
| Journal writing | Writing to another person |
| Critical incident analysis | Writing as the other |
| Dialogical writing | Writing as the journalist |
| Making a case | Storytelling<br>Poetry |

This section uses and expands this classification to provide you with a range of examples and illustrations. Some of these you will already have met – either through the examples already given in this book or because you are required to use them in your course. But others will not be so familiar to you, in fact, you may not even have considered them as useful strategies for reflective writing at all.

### Analytical strategies

These are called analytical strategies because the processes of analysis and synthesis are incorporated within the process of writing. They are the ones that you will meet most commonly because they are amenable to use within the reflective frameworks that have come to dominate reflective practice. They are also likely to use most of the stages of the ERA reflective cycle, although at first the movement to

*Case study continued*

that I might suffer, for example an official reprimand or other disciplinary action. Before I entered the room, I had been confident of my skills and abilities within that environment. I had carried out this procedure hundreds of times before without any significant difficulties. Once this happened, I felt exactly the opposite of this. There was almost a surge of panic flowing through me – while this may have been an over-reaction, it is what I felt, possibly because I had been so confident beforehand.

The patient's reaction to the incident was very good. Indeed, she dealt with it better than I did. I had been speaking with her while the swelling was going down in her hand, and she seemed quite calm. After I had completed my round, I returned to check on her condition, and she seemed to be quite happy. She was sitting with her visitors, laughing and joking. I saw her the next day and asked her how her hand was and she informed me that she had forgotten about the whole episode. This reassured me that her hand was fine and that she suffered no emotional trauma due to this situation.

### Influencing factors

The main internal factor that influenced my actions at the beginning of the incident was my impatience. My biggest concern was that I was held up with the patient and so would not finish my workload early. As it was the weekend and the weather was pleasant, I did not want to spend any more time than was necessary at work. After I had scratched the woman's artery, the factor that influenced my actions was the training I had received beforehand, combined with a new-found sense of urgency arising from the panic that I was experiencing. I also believe that over-confidence was a major contributing factor in my initial actions. I had a fair degree of previous experience and had never had a problem like this one before.

The external factors that were affecting me included the patient and the equipment that I was using to take the blood. The patient had informed me that the back of her hand was the place where other phlebotomists were usually successful at drawing blood. As the woman had been admitted with dehydration, I was inclined to believe her. From past experience, I found that the hand was usually easier to palpate than the crook of the elbow, although research tends to suggest the opposite. The equipment influenced my actions, because the gloves that I was wearing were not suited to the type of work being performed, and so were, in themselves, a contributing factor.

The knowledge base for my actions was the training that I had received during purpose-designed study days, including a practical course in venepuncture. Another source of knowledge for reacting in the way that I did was some basic first-aid knowledge from other courses that I had attended. These courses taught me how to deal with a patient with arterial bleeding. The last source of knowledge was the practical experience that I had in taking venous blood samples. I had been taking blood from patients for over a year with no major difficulties, and had become quite proficient.

### Alternative actions

I believe that I could have dealt with the initial situation better. My actions after the situation had occurred, however, were directly in accordance with the guidelines laid out by that Trust.

My other choices could have included making an attempt to take blood from a different part of the woman's hand or arm. I could also have attempted to palpate the area without gloves on and marked the best area to make an attempt. I do not think that this would have made a significant difference, though. As the lady was dehydrated, it is reasonable to assume that her blood pressure would have been lower than normal. This would suggest that it would have been difficult to feel a pulse in her hand, particularly as this artery was situated below another blood vessel.

*Case study continued*

### Learning

The only reasonable explanation as to my actions was my over-confidence in my abilities combined with my impatience in wanting to finish my shift early. This led to me not giving my full attention to the task at hand. This has led me to develop more patience in my work, and has also developed my attention span by making me think more about what I am doing when performing any procedure.

My feelings about the experience are varied. There is shocked realisation that I was capable of making such a mistake in the first place, as well as the knowledge now that emergencies can happen at any time. I have also experienced a feeling of relief that it has happened, because it has led me to be more careful and pay attention in even the most routine of procedures.

The fact that the only consequence that I suffered was a verbal reprimand confirms to me that I followed the correct course of action. I followed the correct procedures as laid down by the Trust and was therefore covered legally. This shows that the procedures are in place for a reason, and that they should be followed at all times.

### Use of a reflective framework

My overall conclusion is that the use of reflective practice is essential to the delivery of quality care. The above example shows how a formal layout of reflection allows us to look back on what we have done and learn from any outcomes. The main lessons included the correct use of time management and the importance of patience when carrying out all duties in a clinical environment. It has also demonstrated that it is through reflection that procedures change and are improved upon, in this instance the use of gloves in this particular directorate.

*NB. References to published sources have been deleted from the original account*

---

### ⚷ *Keywords*

**Dialogical**
Like a conversation/dialogue

**Hypothetical**
Imaginary/possible

In this account the student clearly identifies how he has arrived at his conclusions in using critical incident analysis through a structured framework. He also acknowledges his learning from the incident and has framed action as a result of this experience. He chose to use a framework, in this case Johns's model of structured reflection, to guide his reflection, and clearly found this useful in helping him to identify his learning and future action.

### Dialogical writing

In **dialogical** writing the writer constructs a **hypothetical** conversation between themselves and another person. This could take the form of a question and answer session, or a developmental dialogue. It is particularly useful where an experience has caused a negative emotional response and the writer needs to be able to stand back from the event and adopt a more analytical and cognitive understanding of the situation. Borton's extended framework is appropriate as a guide for dialogical writing, as it enables the account to be structured through a series of questions. Alternatively, it is useful to create a purpose-made structure for each event, dependent on the learning to be achieved as in the following account.

**Case study**

## Dialogical writing

### What is my previous experience?

I have worked for the last 6 years as a Royal Navy Medical Assistant and after my initial training period I further specialised as a Commando trained medic. This then led me to work almost exclusively with the Royal Marines, providing medical support for them on operations and exercises worldwide. Very often I would be the only medically trained person available for these men and further support from the Medical Officer and other medical staff would be a considerable distance away (if, indeed, they were even in the same country). I would provide this medical cover for up to 150 men in very isolated environments and as such I have had to become a medic competent in being able to work alone, not only in dealing with day to day coughs and colds but also in life-threatening immediate/emergency care such as trauma. I have had to work alone and in isolation from other medical staff, making decisions that have made the difference between life and death.

### Why is this relevant to this incident?

This will hopefully explain why as a first-year student nurse I would be deemed competent enough by my mentor to be entrusted with immediate postoperative nursing care (although I should state that during this period my mentor was within the same nursing bay and was immediately available to me if I encountered any problems).

### What happened?

The patient at the centre of this incident was a 23-year-old lady who was admitted to the ward for a planned surgical incision and drainage of a pilonidal sinus. On admission this lady was in good health and was not suffering any other aliments of any description and her blood pressure was recorded at 118/72 millimetres of mercury (mmHg).

### What does this mean?

Tortora and Grabowski (2003) describe blood pressure as the hydrostatic pressure exerted by blood on the artery walls as it flows through them and break the definition of blood pressure further into systolic blood pressure and diastolic blood pressure. O'Toole (1997) explains systolic pressure as the pressure exerted on the artery walls during systole (ventricular contraction), and in a young adult at rest this will rise to roughly 120mmHg. He goes on to describe diastolic pressure as the pressure on the artery walls during diastole (ventricular relaxation), which would be expected to be around 80mmHg. This gives a normal value of approximately 120/80mmHg for a young adult.

### Go on

With these figures in mind I knew that on admission this patient had a relatively normal blood pressure. However on carrying out an initial check of this lady's

*Case study continued*

baseline observations I was surprised to find that her blood pressure (which I checked manually with a sphygmomanometer and stethoscope) had dropped to 96/62 mmHg. Knowing this patient had just returned to the ward post-operation and from my previous experience I knew that a decreased systolic blood pressure was one of the signs of hypovolaemic shock (Linderman and McAthie 1999).

**So what did I do?**

I wanted to check my patient's blood pressure again to make sure I had not misinterpreted my reading as the ward was busy and very noisy at this time; however, the reading I obtained was the same, so I informed the staff nurse, who immediately checked the patient's blood pressure for herself. The reading she obtained was similar to mine at 98/60mmHg and before contacting the house officer we raised the foot of the bed to help the patient regain a normal blood pressure. On reporting these facts to the house officer (by phone as he was off the ward at the time) he agreed that the patient's blood pressure was lower than normal and he instructed the staff nurse to increase the drip rate of the intravenous infusion, which was still running through postoperatively. He also gave instructions for the staff nurse to inform him immediately if the patient's systolic blood pressure fell below 90mmHg and to check it every 5 minutes for the next 30 minutes and to continue with normal protocols if it began to rise. Thankfully our patient's blood pressure did start to rise and by 2 hours post-operation had returned to almost normal values.

**So what was the problem?**

I was very surprised that the staff nurse felt the need to request further advice from a house officer initially when simple nursing interventions could have improved our patient's blood pressure to the point where normal values might well have been achieved. What did surprise me was that the staff nurse did not act more positively on her own intuition although this could have been due to her own knowledge or experiences.

**Now what sense can I make of this?**

Internally my previous experience had a big effect on my actions, in that as an experienced Royal Navy medic I feel that I am quite competent to check a patient's blood pressure postoperatively. Externally I would have to seriously question my abilities/ knowledge if I was unsure as to what action to take on finding a low blood pressure reading postoperatively given my previous employment. I realise, however, that the staff nurse has not had my experience and has been trained to work in different situations. I realise that I was judging her actions from my own knowledge base, and that this might not have been appropriate. She was responsible for the patient and followed her own reasoning in calling the doctor. Ultimately, it was up to the doctor to prescribe treatment. This was my problem, not hers.

**Now what have I learned from this?**

My main area of learning in light of my previous experience is that I would like to think that as a health-care professional post-registration I will be able to carry out simple but effective and immediate nursing procedures to help improve a patient's outcome. However seeing the staff nurse in this incident request further advice from a house officer before carrying out relatively simple nursing procedures has left me feeling that there are perhaps gaps within pre-registration nurse training. This whole incident has helped me to further my learning by showing me the relevance of checking blood pressure postoperatively, and by using the nursing process nurses can influence patient outcomes for the better. I have also realised that I am perhaps too

*Case study continued*

quick to judge other people, especially as I have a different background from them. In a controlled ward situation I do not have the responsibility that I had in the field and maybe I need to learn to work in a team with the other health-care professionals involved.

**References**

Linderman, C.A. and McAthie, M. (1999) *Fundamentals of Contemporary Nursing Practice*. W.B. Saunders, Philadelphia.

O'Toole, M.T. (ed.) (1997) *Miller-Keane Encyclopedia and Dictionary of Medicine, Nursing and Allied Health*, 6th edn. W.B. Saunders, Philadelphia.

Tortora, G.J. and Grabowski, S.R. (2003) *Principles of Anatomy and Physiology*, 10th edn. John Wiley, New York.

The references have been left in this account to demonstrate how they may be used to support knowledge development, and within evidence based practice.

This was an effective strategy for this reflective account because relatively few cue questions are used yet all stages of the ERA cycle are included. The use of the first person throughout enables the student to sort out his own feelings and responsibilities from those of the other person. It enabled him to let go of his judgement of the staff nurse and focus on the incident in terms of his own learning.

An advantage of this sort of writing is that the dialogue can be led by the writer themselves, in building up a logical sequence. In the account above the stages of the reflective process are all used, but in a way appropriate for the student. For instance, at the stage of exploring alternatives, the student thought about alternative explanations as opposed to alternative actions. His conclusions about the future relate to the way in which he views and assesses other people, and his awareness of making judgements in comparison with himself. His main learning outcome therefore arises not from anything to do with taking blood pressure (he had already recognised his competence in this), nor with the actions of the staff nurse, but from his own attitude to other people and his change of role now he is a student.

**Making a case**

Although similar to dialogical writing, the purpose of this strategy is to create an argument that will persuade another person of the value of the viewpoint presented. This is in many ways very close to an academic writing style, in that you need to present an analysis of a problem, its solutions and your proposals.

## Creative strategies

These strategies are different from the analytical ones because they actively acknowledge the descriptive, personal and emotional components of experiences. In using these strategies, there is a recognition that, at times, we need to get beyond the immediate experience of the event, before we can free ourselves up to explore it analytically and reflectively. Rolfe *et al.* (2001, p. 61) call them creative because they involve 'using the imagination and transforming experience away from the rational ways of analysis which characterises the above group and moves the writer into imagination and metaphor as a way of creating insight and facilitating learning'. The artefact produced may be deliberately one-sided or emphasise the emotionality of the writer's response as opposed to attempting to analyse within the narrative. This serves the purpose of helping the writer to overcome the initial responses to the situation by getting it down on paper in some way. The resulting piece can then be used as the focus for analysis and reflection, or discussion with another person.

It is unlikely that these types of reflective writing would be used in coursework for assessing students. However they may be encouraged in testing out alternative ways of writing in exercises, or be included in students' private reflections on their learning. It would be extremely difficult to justify forcing a student to write in this way because of the vulnerability that can be exposed. It is worth remembering that anyone reading reflective writing will inevitably be making some sort of a judgement about what they are reading, and maybe about the person who has written it too. Indeed, as a student you should never be required to share writing of this kind with others. You are, of course, free to show it of your own volition, but you need to have thought carefully about the consequences of doing so.

### Writing the unsent letter, memo or e-mail

The unsent letter, memo or e-mail all have the same effect – to clear the writer's head of the immediate emotions that accompany a distressing incident. This often occurs when we are angry with someone else or feel that a situation is out of our control, or that we are disempowered in some way.

The idea is that the writer sits and writes exactly what they want to say to the other person involved in the event with no holds barred. Hence, the account may be very emotional, irrational and full of language that you wouldn't actually dream of using to the other person. The safety net is in the fact that the letter/memo/e-mail will not be sent – ever! This is a powerful way of bringing order to the chaos of a stressful situation, and serves the purpose of freeing up the brain to begin dealing with what has occurred. It provides distance from the event itself, yet enables the writer to stay in touch with what happened. Once the writer has got this all down on paper, the account is then used to deconstruct and reflect on what has happened. The result may well be a re-written letter or e-mail that is cleared of the emotionality of the original.

Many of the first accounts from new students resemble this type of work – although this is usually not intentional! For instance, the account below can be seen as an example of reflective writing that should never be made public.

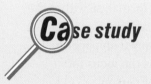

## The unsent letter

Dear Sister

I was really angry at what I saw two trained nurses do today. Victor, an 86-year-old postoperative patient, had an extreme reaction to the anaesthetic and had been vomiting in his bed. Sarah, the staff nurse, decided that he needed a nasogastric tube to relieve the pressure in his stomach. He had been left in a bed covered in vomit and appeared exhausted and upset. She left me with him while she went to get the equipment to pass the tube.

The tube was passed easily but I noticed that Victor was very anxious and put this down to the pain and discomfort he was feeling. Once in place the fluid was expected to drain from the tube, but this didn't happen, probably because the tube wasn't far enough into the stomach. Victor vomited, causing the tube to come out of his mouth. Sarah left the bay for another tube and to get more help. All the staff were busy, and as a result Victor was left lying in vomit for 10 minutes waiting for the next shift to arrive. He looked completely exhausted and traumatised by the whole incident. Then it was decided that the nasogastric tube could wait until the following morning.

Due to the shift overlap handover, both nurses decided to change Victor's pyjamas swiftly. I was told to go off shift as I could be of no further use, but before doing so I noticed both nurses remove the pyjama top and replace it with a clean one without giving Victor a wash. No bathing, clean bed linen or mouth care was offered at all.

I felt absolutely dreadful at Victor's treatment, and pretty disgusted at the standards of care that I have witnessed on this ward. If these are the standards that you allow then I feel you should not be in charge. I certainly do not want to learn how to be a nurse from these qualified staff.

This was obviously a shocking incident as witnessed by a new student on her first placement. It clearly challenged her beliefs and values about nursing, the care that patients can expect to receive and her faith in her mentor as a practitioner. Writing the incident down in his way enabled her to pour out her feelings and emotions so that she could then stand back from the incident. However, to make the incident public in this way would cause a great many more problems for the student than it would solve. Hence she needed to reflect on what she had written and think about her own learning from the incident, and the implications for her future practice, rather than on the actions of the others involved. This is her analytical and reflect account.

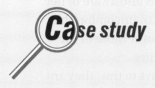

### Victor's treatment – a reflective account

Reflecting back on the incident I feel annoyed and upset that I didn't do more at the time. This was my first ward and only my first week, which made me very unsure of my knowledge and expertise learned previously at the university. I lacked confidence, resulting in a breakdown of my communication skills. When Sarah left the bedside I am embarrassed to say I went numb, unable to speak. I just couldn't find any words appropriate to the situation and to comfort Victor.

When it came to the hygiene aspects of the incident I should have agreed to help but was unsure of how the nurses would react if I suggested a complete washdown and thorough changing of bedding and clothing. I was concerned with what and how they might feel towards me if I were to intervene.

### Good points

It was very difficult at first to see any good points. I valued the educational input from Sarah. I have found the whole experience of reflecting on the incident an excellent learning tool and will use it in the future.

### Bad points

Overall, there appears to be more negative points than positive ones. My communication skills appear lacking, which led to a breakdown in the nurse–patient relationship, resulting in an unprofessional standard of care. I feel that the patient was not central during the situation as his feelings were not considered throughout.

### Analysis

Looking back over the incident I can now see why things turned out the way they did. Communication broke down between nurse and patient, and me and the nurse. Sarah and I were caught up in the teaching and learning aspect and were not concentrating on communicating with Victor. I later learned that Victor is hard of hearing. He must have been feeling very isolated, alone and confused as a result, which is why he got so distressed. Victor had also been given intramuscular metoclopramide to prevent nausea and vomiting. This can cause drowsiness, restlessness and depression – all shown by Victor at the time.

The problem with the insertion of the tube could have been avoided had Sarah measured the approximate distance from nose to stomach.

Victor's capacity to look after his own hygiene needs were severely restricted, and he was unable to wash himself, change his clothes or his bedding. It was the nurses' responsibility to do this.

### Conclusion

Overall I feel that I should have been more assertive and got involved, despite my lack of experience. This does not excuse the overlooking of what should have been basic nursing care. If this situation happened again I would ensure that I communicated effectively with the patient and put his needs before my own. I would also ensure that I left the patient in a clean and comfortable condition, no matter whether that meant I was late going off shift.

**⊶ᴛ *Keywords***

**Portfolio**
A collection of documents
that provides evidence of
your achievements and
professional development

**Selecting your own models and frameworks, or adapting those given to you to suit yourself**  Part of being successful as a reflective writer is that you are able to select from the array of models and structures available, or even to create your own to suit your particular purpose at the time.

**Retaining control over who sees your writing and what they see**  It is essential that you control the product of the writing. It is up to you to decide who, if anybody, sees your writing – no-one can force you to show what you have written to others. Your first ventures into reflective writing for others may be in classwork, for course assignments or for creating your **portfolio**. Despite the interpretations that are often put on these, no-one dictates the content of your writing – you can make choices as to what to use in all of these as the subject of your reflective activity, in illustration or evidence that you have achieved the requirements of, for instance, learning outcomes or criteria for the professional body.

**Storing your writing safely**  Do think about where you will keep your reflective writing once you have done it. Does it need to be in a secret place so that no-one else can access it? Or do you need simply to ensure that it goes into a folder out of the way? If you are writing on computer, does anyone else have access to it, and would it bother you if they read what you had written? One student went as far as only saving his work to a floppy disk and storing this in a locked cupboard to prevent others having access to his reflections. You may not have this kind of need for secrecy and security, but giving thought to who might accidentally see your work and planning to avoid this will give you more freedom in what you write and how you write it.

**Planning to complete the reflective cycle**  The success of writing reflectively, as with any other reflective activity that you will meet in this book, is that of completing the reflective cycle. It is often not the subject, or the content, of what you reflect on that is necessarily important, but its analysis in terms of what can be drawn out in understanding and learning. Writing reflectively is simply one way of doing this – one tool in the kit bag – which will suit some people and not others, just as many of the techniques throughout the book will have more appeal to some of us than others.

> ### 👉 *Over to you*
>
> It is clearly up to you who sees your work, and what you choose to do with it. However, these need to be conscious decisions that are taken thoughtfully, if you are to have the safety to write of your own experiences, reactions to them and feelings about them. Developing insight about ourselves is an illuminating and educating process and can bring great satisfaction. It is also risky and can be threatening; therefore we owe it to ourselves to ensure that we minimise risks.
>
> What can you do to ensure that you are safe in your reflective writing?

### *Key points*  Top tips

- There are a variety of analytical and creative strategies and styles for reflective writing that can be used to work through the ERA cycle
- Any of these can be used with a structured framework for reflection
- It is not, however, necessary to use a structured framework for writing reflectively
- Writing is a purposive and deliberate activity that helps to provide different insights into our experiences
- We can take control of our writing and create strategies ourselves for writing safely.

## Using reflective writing within a portfolio

The aim of this section is to explore ways in which you can incorporate the reflective work that you do within a portfolio. This is intended only as an introduction to the ideas behind portfolio construction and to give you a few pointers to help you. More detailed advice and information, as well as a CD providing a portfolio template, will be found in another book in this series: *Profiles and Portfolios of Evidence* by Ruth Pearce (2003).

Many health-care professions now ask qualified practitioners to keep a record of their continuing professional development as a requirement for periodic registration. In preparation for this, health-care students are likely to begin starting their portfolios as part of their course. Other students may meet portfolios during their course for recording their practice, or as part of the coursework that they do. These are usually aimed at enabling the student to recognise their unique and individual development and learning as opposed to the more generic work that they do using other forms of assessment.

Hence, the experiences that you gain of portfolio work as a student will be setting you up for the professional portfolio that you will need to keep once you are qualified. Some of the contents within your portfolio will be your reflective work, which shows how you are applying your knowledge and learning from the experiences that you have in practice.

## What is a portfolio?

A portfolio is traditionally seen as a collection of documents that provides a picture to a third party of what that person is like. For instance, an artist might have a portfolio of his work that shows his style and type of work; or a government minister might have a portfolio that outlines her area of responsibility. More recently, the concept of a portfolio has developed within professional practice in terms of documenting and providing evidence of the practitioner's continuing competence and development. This is a movement away from the portfolio as being purely a record of things that have happened to a continuously changing artefact that is used for learning. In this context, the most commonly found definition of a portfolio is that of Brown (1992), who says that a personal portfolio is:

> *a private collection of evidence which demonstrates the continuing acquisition of skills, knowledge, attitudes and achievement.*
> *It is both retrospective and prospective, as well as reflecting the current stage of development and activity of the individual.*

Portfolios are used by students in learning contexts to build a collection of evidence. This evidence demonstrates that they are making progress towards achieving the learning outcomes that are expected of them. So the portfolio is constructed for a particular purpose, as opposed to having free content decided by the student. The kinds of document we see in portfolios might include:

- A learning contract
- A list of the learning outcomes that are to be achieved in the course, module or practice placement
- A list of clinical/practical competencies that need to be achieved
- Plans for action for achieving the outcomes and competencies
- Reflective reviews of experience
- Self-assessment documents
- Evidence that demonstrates achievements
- Contributions from other people that support the claims being made
- Your learning journal or diary
- Personal sections in the portfolio that will not necessarily be shown to other people.

Other things that might be included if you are maintaining a general portfolio from which you select specific items for different purposes might be:

- Your CV
- Your previous job descriptions
- Placement descriptions and what you learned within them
- Any special skill development
- Any achievements or special awards
- Your certificates.

You might also want to include material from other people that supports the claims that you are making. Examples might be:

- Letters that mention your work
- Statements from supervisors or others you have worked with
- Copies of programmes for study days or conferences you have attended
- Reports from clinical practice in which you are mentioned
- Evidence that prove that you were a part of something that happened.

This kind of portfolio is essentially a public document because it is being constructed for a specific purpose and is a requirement of a course. Therefore, students need to make decisions about what the portfolio is going to say to the outside world about them, and the kind of picture it will be presenting. It can be compared to compiling a family photograph album. When we choose from all the pictures that we have, we want to select those that present the best possible picture of us. We are unlikely to show others unflattering shots or ones that we would be embarrassed about – unless that is specifically what we want to do, of course! So, actively selecting from what we have available to go into the portfolio is very important in creating this picture of ourselves.

### Selecting the material for a portfolio

As a student it is likely that a format for the portfolio, and what you are expected to put into it, will be decided for you. But within this, you still have a great deal of leeway in deciding what, from all of your work, will present the best picture of you. Some of this will be the reflective accounts that you have constructed through the course. Other work to include might be reflections of what you have done independently and want to include in the portfolio because you feel it demonstrates your learning and development.

When you are with friends, or even in a working relationship, it is easy to slip into talking over events and things that have happened. You'll probably be more aware of this at the outset of any reflective activity that you do with your mentor/supervisor and your educational advisors. Encounters with the last two groups are likely to be more formal, planned and focused on outcomes that are predefined. These may be about identifying your learning as a result of work you have done in placement, and end up in defining what more you need to achieve, or follow up on. They might also be about your progress so far, how you are doing against set criteria for the placement, and planning for the rest of your time there. Yet another type of reflective event may be specifically about an incident that has happened, where you spend time exploring what has occurred, to learn from it and so that you can take this forward as one of your own paradigm cases.

Similarly, in an educational setting, the chances are that lecturers will focus on what they want you to achieve as a result of the reflective work. But, this doesn't stop you thinking about it beforehand and planning your own objectives and outcomes. This is particularly so if you have a one-to-one tutorial that has a time limit to it and there are specific things that you want to know about or achieve. Lecturers are usually busy people and need to make the most of tutorial time. They will appreciate you spending a little time thinking through what you want from the tutorial and coming along armed with a list, and pen and paper to make notes as you go along. This can be especially important if you are asking for advice on assignments coming up that you have queries about. It is easy to sit and think 'I'll remember that' and then get outside and realise that you haven't taken in a word that was said! It is also worth writing up your tutorials and using them as a focus for reflection, in terms of capitalising on your learning from others and the communication strategies that you develop in negotiating with educational staff.

All three types of encounter will have more benefit if you plan what it is you want out of them before you start. This needn't take long, but setting a few goals to focus your mind and planning to achieve outcomes makes the most effective use of your time, and the other person's. Similarly, writing up the event in your learning journal provides you with the time to think things over and create a record. In particular, getting into the habit of concisely identifying what you feel you have learned each day provides an on-going record of your progress and development.

So, here are a few useful tips to think about before embarking on reflective sessions with someone else.

- Establish the purpose of the encounter with the other person at the outset
- Be aware of what you are saying and the implications that this might have
- Think about setting boundaries/rules of engagement/outcomes
- Be prepared to accept that others may have different views from you and that these are not only valid but worthy of consideration
- Be aware of what you are asking the other person to do – either as the person reflecting on an experience or as another person in the reflective relationship.

## The nature of the relationship

The nature of the relationship you have with the person will have an effect on several aspects of the event. The types of people you will be working with fall into three main groups:

- Friends, peers, colleagues, partners and family
- Professional workers – your mentor/supervisor or assessor, other workers in your own discipline and members of other professions
- Educational staff – your lecturers, link tutors in clinical placements, your personal tutor, etc.

Clearly, you will have a different sort of relationship with the people in each of these groups, and this will affect the type of reflective work that you do with them. Three issues are of particular importance here.

### Issues of trust

Being able trust the people that you reflect with is of crucial importance if you are going to be able to learn from the work you do. This can take many forms. First of all, you need to feel comfortable with the person, whether that means that you appear to be on the same wavelength, that you talk the 'same language', that you feel they will not be judgemental or that they allow you the space to talk without interrupting. Secondly, you need to have faith in the other person's judgement; consider whether you think they can offer sound advice that is in your own best interests and whether they have the information, knowledge and experience that you need. Finally, perhaps you need to consider the other person's interpersonal skills and how they communicate with you. Do they truly listen and empathise with you and are they able to reflect back to you in a caring way, helping you come to a different understanding of your situation?

### Confidentiality

Another way in which we need to be able to trust people that we reflect with is to be reassured that the conversation is private and that elements of it will not be spread around to others. This is a difficult issue, because very often we do not think that we need to say 'This is just between you and me' or 'I would not want anyone else to know about this'. This is especially so when it is our friends that we are talking with and we take it as read that we can trust them in this way.

However, the boundaries are not so clear when it comes to reflecting in a professional capacity, as your mentor or tutor may feel that the issue is of wider concern and they need to consult with other people. Take Heidi's experience, for instance. As a result of your talk with her, she might have decided to go to her tutor at college and talk about her problem. In turn, the tutor may decide that s/he needs to intervene in the student/mentor relationship, as there are clearly problems here that need resolving if Heidi is to have a successful learning experience under Ben's mentorship.

The implications here are that clear boundaries need to be set from the beginning of any reflective activity with other people. If, at the start of a conversation you clearly state that what you are going to say is of a delicate nature and at this time you do not want it to go any further than the people in the room, then they have to opportunity to say whether or not they can abide by that. It is up to them to say if they are not prepared to play the game by your rules. If they have reservations and feel that they may need to take something further, then you also have the option of not sharing with them what you were going to say, and seeking out a different forum. Similarly, of course, if you are the one in the listening seat, you need to consider your own commitment to confidentiality, and whether you are able to keep other people's confidences to yourself. Some people find it difficult to keep secrets or, with the best will in the world, may inadvertently act on information that has been received in confidence. If you know that your best friend, or the tutor that you talk to, has a tendency to do this, you have the choice of talking to them or not. If you know that you find it difficult not to use information, or to keep a confidence, it is only fair to the person talking to you to say this and allow them to make the decision about whether or not to carry on.

The issue of confidentiality also arises when talking about other people, in particular where patients and clients are involved, or other ward staff. As a student in a professional capacity, you have a responsibility to respect the confidentiality of others and not to make information about them public. So, if you are planning to use your experiences with patients as the basis for reflective work, do ensure that anything you use is anonymous and is not likely to identify the person concerned.

### Assessment

Many of the people that you reflect with will also be acting as your assessors in some way. This includes, not only people who will formally assess you by marking your work or completing your practical assessment documents, but also to those you work with, and other lecturers, who will be feeding in to the overall assessment of you during your course. Anyone who is responsible for assessing you has a dual role. Not only will they be guiding and teaching you throughout the time you are with them but they will also be making judgements about you, your learning and your competence to practise. At the end of the day, it is your assessors who approve your licence to practise; it is their judgement that determines whether you will qualify as a professional practitioner or not. This means that sometimes it is worth being cautious about with whom you choose to reflect, and what it is you disclose to them.

Identifying the nature of the relationship that you have with the people you choose to reflect with is important in planning for your reflective activity to be successful. Remember that everyone is not there to be your friend – they all have their own professional roles and responsibilities in interacting with you, and this will determine the kind of the interaction that you have with them. Acknowledging this and planning to use this in a positive sense is crucial in ensuring that you enter a reflective relationship feeling secure and able to trust that person. Thinking about this in advance and planning the interaction that you have will help you to feel that you have some control, as will negotiating the boundaries for the interaction and the ground rules under which it continues.

## Setting boundaries and ground rules for reflecting with others

This sounds a rather formal and intimidating step to take. In reality, once you get used to doing this it not only ensures that both you and the other person have a clear understanding of what it is that you are there to do, it also helps you to use your time effectively and achieve what you want from the encounter.

### Time and place

There are some basic elements to this that might sound obvious. First of all, think about what kind of environment and setting you will feel happiest and most relaxed in. Being clear about the time that you are going to meet, the amount of time that you will spend reflecting with the other person and where you will do this clearly establishes the activity as a formal appointment with some purpose. It will signal a commitment from both of you and acknowledge that there is serious work to be done – you are not just turning up for a chat!

Choosing a place to work in has a dramatic effect on how relaxed you will feel, how secure and safe you will be and to what extent you are able to settle into a conversation. A review of your progress with your assessor, for instance, is not likely to be confidential if it is carried out in an office that has open access to other people, with phones ringing and others working at desks. You are unlikely to feel confident in this sort of environment about discussing issues that you feel should be kept between the two of you. Developing assertive skills here, by suggesting a more appropriate environment prior to the meeting, avoids any problems of this sort on the day.

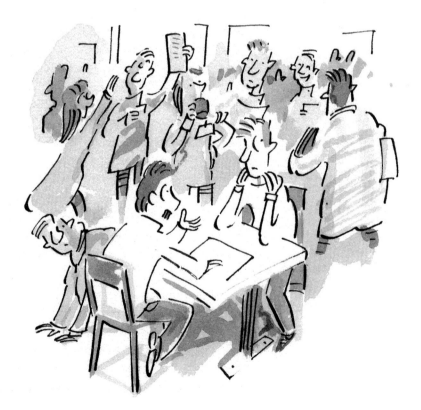

*You should always insist on a suitable setting for your reflective meetings*

### Setting the focus of the meeting

Again, if the focus of the meeting is negotiated in advance it allows both sides in the encounter the chance to plan and gather information. This might simply be that you ensure you have notes about the issue before you attend the meeting, and that you have already reflected by yourself on what it is that you want to achieve by the end. It also gives the other person an idea of what the issue or issues may be and they can ensure that they have the relevant information, documentation, etc. so that the most is made of the time available.

The other person may have initiated the meeting and have their own agenda – again, if you can have a part of this it enables you to feel that you have some control in the encounter and that you are valued as an equal in the process. For instance, if you have booked a tutorial to talk about a draft assignment, it is important that you have submitted it in good time to allow your tutor to have read it and made comments. Turning up with the assignment in your hand is unfair – your tutor cannot give you adequate feedback while reading the work in front of you. However, if you have got it to them in advance, it is reasonable on your part to assume that they will have read it and will be able to use the time effectively in feedback.

### Identifying the meeting's outcomes

Managing the content and focus of reflective meetings in this way ensures that you focus on the issue identified and that you are setting up the meeting to be effective. The next thing to think about is what it is that you want to achieve as a result of the meeting.

One of the most satisfying aspects of reflecting with other people is that you can plan to come up with some answers and some action as a result of the encounter, when you might not be able to do so by yourself. Some meetings will have easily definable outcomes, such as identifying further library work that you want to do in order to understand the theory behind something you have encountered in practice. At other times, however, it is not so simple. Often, we go into reflective activities with others without having envisaged a tangible outcome. We might think things like 'I just want to know what to do' or 'I want to get this sorted out'. Well, this is as good a place as any to start. Turning these into outcomes that you can phrase in an objective way starts the reflective process and enables you to start stepping back from the situation and creating a distance between you and the event. If it is possible for you to do this before the meeting, and go into it with clearly defined objectives, then you have already done a lot of the work.

However, it is not essential to do this; what is essential is that you start off the meeting by exploring with the other person what it is that you, and they, want to achieve.

**Managing the meeting**

You also have to consider, however, how the meeting will work. Ground rules for the meeting itself, and the parts that the people play within it, bear some thinking about. When there are only two of you in the meeting, it may be important that the balance of the conversation is skewed in one direction, depending on the meeting's focus and intention. Issues that you might like to consider are:

- How both people will be able to say what they want to say in safety
- The type of language that you will use
- How you will manage confidentiality
- What role you will each play in the meeting
- How you determine the action that both people will take as a result of the meeting
- How you will record the meeting.

This probably all sounds very complicated, and you may be wondering if it is all worth it in the end. Let's face it, not all meetings that you have will work like this. You will not be in the position of being able to think through these processes and get everything sorted out in your mind in this way every time you plan to meet up with another person for reflective activity. But, equally, there will be occasions where you are able to do this, and it is worth taking 5 minutes or so beforehand to ensure that you make the most effective use of your time with the other person. Taking responsibility for your own learning is the key to reflective practice. A conscious use of the processes of learning from reflection will enable you to achieve your outcomes more quickly and effectively than simply waiting for things to happen!

**Key points** Top tips

- Choose the time and place to suit the type of encounter, and keep to them!
- Identify the focus of the meeting and negotiate what both parties will do in preparation for it
- Write down what you want to achieve from the meeting and negotiate with the other person what they want to get out of it
- Talk about confidentiality at the start of the meeting if this is appropriate
- Agree ground rules about the way the meeting is conducted

## Considering the risks of reflecting with others

What does this mean? In any encounter with another person there will be risks involved. When using reflection as a tool to learn from experience, there is always a range of outcomes that may occur because the subject of the reflection is, in the majority of cases, something that has happened to you, which means that you have an emotional stake in the experience. Although the focus of any reflective activity can come from the whole range of your experiences, often it is those that have left you feeling uncomfortable, or where you are unhappy with the outcome, that are the subject of your reflective activity. These, then, also have the potential to cause us more stress because they have arisen from situations in which we have felt vulnerable and out of control. For instance:

- You might not like what others say to you
- You might feel uncomfortable with the 'reflective mirror' that others hold up to you
- You may feel overpowered or taken in directions that you do not feel comfortable with
- You may feel that others are judging you
- You may feel that you are under attack
- You may feel that you have done something wrong
- You may feel that you lack control in the encounter.

Anticipating the risks of a reflective encounter helps to prepare you for what you may experience. Probably the most important way of doing this is to use the stages of the process outlined in the previous sections to move your perception of the meeting from focusing on something that you have done to a chance to learn from experience. Creating a distance from the focus of the encounter helps us to use the experience of others to maximum effect. In particular, negotiating ground rules for conducting the meeting is vital to avoid situations such as those described above; learning is unlikely to occur if you feel threatened and attacked by what happens during the meeting.

**Key points** | Top tips

- Use the ground rules previously negotiated to keep the conduct of the meeting fair and equitable to all
- Use the meeting's facilitator (in a group situation) if you feel under threat
- Be clear in stating to the group/other person if you feel unhappy about what is happening
- Focus on the outcomes that you want to achieve
- Never ask a question that you don't really want an answer to, or if you haven't prepared yourself for an answer that you weren't expecting
- Try to end the encounter on a positive note

## The professional and/or ethical implications

All health-care professionals work within professional codes of conduct and ethics, whether formal or informal. An example of a code of principles is that of the Nursing and Midwifery Council (2002), which states:

*As a professional nurse or midwife, you are personally accountable for your practice.*

*In caring for patients and clients, you must:*

- *Respect the patient or client as an individual*
- *Obtain consent before you give any treatment or care*
- *Protect confidential information*
- *Co-operate with others in the team*
- *Maintain your professional knowledge and competence*
- *Be trustworthy*
- *Act to identify and minimise risk to patients and clients.*

Nursing and Midwifery Council (2002), available at www.nmc-uk.org

This code has been accepted by all health-care professions as incorporating the basic principles for their practice. The Health Professions Council, formed in 2003, brings together the previously separate professions allied to medicine for registration and regulatory purposes. Part of its area of responsibility is to ensure that all health-care professions work within an established code of conduct incorporating standards for practice and ethical guidelines.

Therefore, it is important to remember that, whenever you are reflecting with other people in a professional capacity (even with other students), you must be aware of the responsibilities that you and the other person have according to the code of conduct. Many of the events that you reflect upon and use as the focus for reflective encounters with other people will be incidents that have caused you to be uncomfortable in some way. These might involve what you consider to be unsatisfactory standards of care given to patients or clients; misconduct or negligence by another member of staff; abuse of patients, particularly vulnerable people such as children, the elderly or people with learning disabilities; or episodes of care that you consider to be ethically suspect.

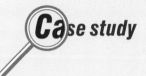

## Case study

### Jim is an unwilling witness

Jim was working with Mrs W on Buttercup Ward, assessing her swallowing after she had had a stroke. He became aware of raised voices in the single room next door and couldn't help hearing what was going on. The nurse was trying to change the dressings on Mr T's legs. This was not an easy or pleasant task for either of them because his leg ulcers were extensive and had an unpleasant-smelling exudate that dried between dressings, making them very difficult to remove. Mr T hated having his dressings done because it was very painful. The nurses gave him painkillers before the procedure, and offered him gas and air during the worst bits.

On this occasion though it was obvious that things weren't going right. Mr T was telling the nurse that she wasn't doing it right, and to leave him alone. The nurse seemed to lose her temper, called him an ungrateful old man and said that she was going to do what she had to. She then gave him a few home truths, which, as an unwilling witness, Jim found embarrassing. He wasn't sure what happened next, but he heard what sounded like someone being hit. Mr T grunted and it all went very quiet. A few minutes later the nurse came out of the room, and Jim looked in to see if Mr T was all right. He noticed what looked like a fresh bruise on Mr T's face.

### Reflective activity

What should Jim do next?

Imagine you were the one that witnessed this happening, and decided to use it as the focus for a reflective tutorial with your tutor.

- What would you want to achieve from the tutorial?
- What are the implications within your professional code of conduct in terms of:
  - Your responsibility towards the patient concerned
  - Your responsibility towards the nurse
  - Your professional responsibility as a student practitioner in maintaining standards and ensuring patient safety
  - Confidentiality?
- What responsibility did Jim's supervisor have on hearing the story?
- What might be the implications for the tutor that you are discussing it with?

In sharing issues of this kind with other people, you must be aware that action might need to be taken as a result of what you have said. This can be extremely difficult for all concerned, and it is vital that you consider these issues before deciding to talk to others about incidents with an element of professional misconduct. Other registered practitioners have a duty, as do you, to report any incident where standards of care and the professional code of conduct are breached.

You may not have witnessed such an incident but may actually have done something that contravenes the code of conduct. We need to bear the code of professional conduct in mind all the time and attempt to achieve professionally acceptable standards of behaviour in everything we do. This includes:

- The ways in which we speak to and of other people
- The type of language we use with others
- The ways in which we act in the clinical environment
- The ways in which we treat other people
- The consideration we give to respecting others and maintaining their dignity at all times
- Attempting to do our patients and clients no harm
- Acting in the patients' best interests at all times
- The impression that we give others when we are not in the clinical environment, e.g. the message that others may get if they see a nurse smoking when in uniform

as well as the more clinical or practical elements of our job.

**Key points** Top tips

When considering reflecting with others in a professional context, think about:
- The contextual implications of discussing things that have happened
- Choosing what to tell and considering the implications of this
- Working within professional codes of conduct and discuss the implications of this
- The consequences of disclosure
- Misconduct/malpractice/negligence
- Understanding the responsibilities of others within their professional role

# Contexts for reflecting with others

Finally, we need to think about the context in which we reflect with other people. First of all, we will consider the issues to be considered when you are engaging in reflective work with one other person, and when you will be part of a group using reflective techniques for learning. Secondly we want to look at the differing issues involved when you are reflecting with the three groups of people who have a part in your education.

## Reflecting in a one-to-one relationship

There are two primary relationships that occur when you are reflecting with one other person. First, there is the informal relationship that you have with your peers, colleagues, fellow students, friends and relatives. Second, there is the more formal type of relationship that you have with your supervisor, other professional colleagues and your academic tutors.

The nature of the relationship you have with members of each of these groups is, by necessity, different – the only reason that you have a relationship with the second group is because you are a student.

---

### *Reflective activity*

**Reflecting on a one-to-one basis has certain benefits**

What might these benefits be?

What might the disadvantages be?

---

In preparing for any reflective activity with another person in a one-to-one relationship, we can summarise the issues as:

- Setting ground rules and boundaries; contracts
- Establishing purposes and outcomes
- Defining responsibilities
- Framing action.

## Reflecting in a group

You are likely to find yourself reflecting as a group within two main contexts. Most probably, you will use group work in an educational setting, facilitated by a lecturer or practitioner. However, you may also find yourself in a group in the practice environment, as more and more clinical areas establish reflective practice techniques in the workplace for continual professional development. Some areas may do this specifically for all the students in their specialty.

Reflecting in a group is an extremely valuable way of broadening your perspective on an issue, as you will meet with others whose views are not known to you and who can bring entirely different experiences into the group. However, while working reflectively in groups has benefits, again, there are issues about the dynamics of groups, and the risks inherent in several people being involved, that need to be thought through.

---

## *Reflective activity*

What will be different about reflecting in a group from reflecting with just one person?

How can you plan to use these features effectively to maximise your learning?

---

Some of the issues you may have thought about are:

- Who is facilitating the group, and what are their roles and responsibilities
- Establishing the ground rules and boundaries for the life of the group
- Establishing the commitment of the group members
- Ensuring you feel safe – this relates to what you are prepared to say in the group setting and who you are prepared to say it to
- Agreeing rules for confidentiality
- Identifying the purpose of the group
- Identifying the learning that has been achieved
- Framing action as a result on both a group and personal basis.

### Reflecting with peers, colleagues and friends

When you can choose the person that you talk to, maybe a friend, another student or a member of your family, you have a large element of control within the encounter and are likely to feel safer and more secure in the way you talk to them. With these people you have a complex set of relationships that change with the different roles you are in. These informal relationships enable you to take a very different

**○━┯ *Keywords***

**Tripartite**
Involving three people

approach to reflection with another person from when you are in a working relationship with them. As a result, the reflecting you do is likely to be less formal and less structured. You may find that you rarely use a framework for reflection with these people, unless you specifically set out to do so.

---

## Reflective activity

What might be the advantages of reflecting with someone with whom you have a friendship, relationship, or informal acquaintance?

What might the drawbacks be?

How can you use these to reflect effectively with this group of people?

---

### Using mentors/assessors and clinical supervision

Similarly, reflecting with this group of people will have its own character. These people are not only in a professional relationship with you and have certain responsibilities towards you in that capacity, they are also members of a profession themselves and therefore act as gatekeepers for that profession. Hence, the reflective work you do with them will be more formal in its nature, and probably directed at achieving specific purposes.

---

## Reflective activity

Think again about the benefits that these features bring to the reflective encounters.

What issues will you need to think about before this type of activity?

---

These last two activities are really asking you to review what you have learned from the previous sections of this chapter and apply it to yourself.

The contexts in which you may be reflecting with this group of people are:

- Establishing your learning needs at the beginning of a placement
- Clinical supervision/formal reflective sessions throughout the placement
- Reflective reviews of your learning
- **Tripartite** meetings with your supervisor and link teacher

- Informal reflective sessions
- Seizing the moment (reflecting in action/on the hoof)
- Talking after the action (reflection on action)
- Seeking others out in response to things that have happened
- Bouncing ideas around

### Using academic staff

Finally, we turn to your relationship with the academic staff. Again, this relationship has a different nature and context from those involving the other groups of people.

---

## Reflective activity

What are the special features of your relationship with academic staff?

How do these differ from those you have with others?

How can you plan to use these features in working reflectively with academic staff?

---

All the academic staff that you work with will have several functions within their relationship with you. Some of these are:

- As a teacher
- As a facilitator
- As a personal tutor
- As a confidante
- As a clinical tutor/link lecturer
- As a marker/assessor of your work and progress
- As a professional gatekeeper
- As a maintainer of standards
- As a supporter.

Their primary role may be to support you in your learning throughout your course. But they also have professional responsibilities belonging to their roles as an employee of an academic institution and as a member of their profession. These two roles both carry a responsibility for upholding standards, and this is bound up within the relationship they have with you. As a result, any reflective work you do with them will be framed within these three functions.

tɔɘlʇɘЯ*Reflective activity*

In this last activity, we want you to think about the types of reflective encounter that you might have with academic staff. Use the list of the lecturer's functions above as a focus.

What might you want to achieve from these?

How can you plan to use these to your advantage?

Within all these contexts, each person in the relationship has their own agenda and responsibilities. Your primary roles as a student will be in ensuring that you are using the reflective processes involved to learn and develop towards being a professional practitioner. While these will certainly be a part of the intentions of the others involved, they will also have different purposes for the activities. Therefore, it is up to you to think about each encounter in advance and plan to achieve what it is you need. This may even involve taking some sort of control during the meeting to ensure that your needs are met as well as the other person's. It always helps if you plan in advance, and maybe even go along with a list of the things that you want to achieve as a guide for the time that you have available. This will help you to make the most of this and ensures you maximise your learning.

**Key points** Top tips

- We can use the different relationships that we have with others for different kinds of reflection
- One-to-one reflection has a different nature from group reflection
- Forward planning before any reflective encounter with others will ensure that our own needs are met
- Remember that every person involved in a reflective relationship has differing needs from it and will be working to achieve these
- The primary responsibility for the student's learning within reflective encounters lies with the student.

## Conclusions

Throughout this chapter we have tried to take a balanced view of the advantages and challenges of reflecting with other people. This is clearly different from reflecting by yourself. While it brings huge rewards in helping you to see different perspectives and think about your experiences in different ways, it also carries certain risks and vulnerabilities with it that need active management and forward planning.

As with all reflective activity, the more you think about what you want to achieve by reflecting with other people, the more you are likely to get from it. By identifying the learning outcomes so that you are able to take some sort of action, you will be completing the ERA cycle every time. As a result, you will be functioning as a reflective practitioner in all the contexts in which you operate.

---

## RRRRR Rapid recap

Check your progress so far by working through each of the following questions.

1. What are the benefits of reflecting with others?
2. What different groups of people could you choose to reflect with?
3. What issues do you need to think about before starting to reflect with others?
4. How can you make the most of reflecting with others?

If you have difficulty with more than one of the questions, read through the section again to refresh your understanding before moving on.

---

## References

Nursing and Midwifery Council (2002) *The Professional Code of Conduct*. NMC, London.

## Further reading

We have not gone into a lot of detail about clinical supervision here, but this is clearly an area where reflective practice is encouraged and developed. The following sources will provide you with further understanding of it.

Fisher, M. (1996) Using reflective practice in clinical supervision. *Professional Nurse* **11** 443–444.

Fitzgerald, M. (2000) Clinical supervision and reflective practice. In: Bulman C and Burns S (eds) *Reflective Practice in Nursing*, 2nd edn. Oxford: Blackwell Scientific.

Rolfe, G., Freshwater, D. and Jasper, M. (2001) *Critical Reflection for Nursing and the Helping Professions: A user's guide*. Basingstoke: Palgrave.
This book has two chapters about clinical supervision, which provide a useful outline of the principles of both individual and group supervision.

# Appendix

# Rapid Recap – answers

## Chapter 1

1.  **What is the ERA cycle of reflective practice?**
    Experience–reflection–action

2.  **What are Schön's two types of reflection?**
    Reflection-in-action and reflection-on-action

3.  **What is the difference between the reflective processes and reflective practice?**
    Reflective practice requires some sort of action to be taken

4.  **What are the stages in the reflective processes?**
    The stages of the reflective processes are:
    Stage 1: Selecting a critical incident to reflect on
    Stage 2: Observing and describing the experience
    Stage 3: Analysing the experience
    Stage 4: Interpreting the experience
    Stage 5: Exploring alternatives.
    Stage 6: Framing action

5.  **What is meant by the term 'critical incident'?**
    A critical incident is an event that stands out in your mind and contributes directly to developing as a practitioner

## Chapter 2

1.  **What is a SWOB analysis?**
    A SWOB analysis is a way of identifying your strengths and weaknesses, the opportunities that you have and the barriers to achieving these

2.  **Where do our professional values come from?**
    Professional values come from a variety of sources including:
    Received from external sources – media, people we know, careers information
    Our own personality, attitudes and approach to life, and cultural experiences
    Other professionals
    Generally accepted beliefs and moral codes
    Codes of professional conduct

3.  **How can knowing your preferred learning style help you to learn more effectively?**
    Recognising the ways in which we learn helps us to select methods that we will benefit from most

4.  **What are the challenges to using writing to learn?**
    Challenges might be:
    - Overcoming the rules for writing
    - Writing for ourselves instead of others
    - Using the features of the 'writing-to-learn' paradigm
    - Overcoming the need to 'get it right'
    - Completing the reflective cycle
    - Deciding on the difference between public and private writing
    - Anticipating the consequences of our writing
    - Finding something to write about
    - Getting started

## Chapter 3

1. **What are Goodman's three levels of reflection?**

   First level – reflection to reach given objectives

   Second level – reflection on the relationship between principles and practice

   Third level – reflection that, besides the above, incorporates ethical and political concerns

2. **What are the six stages of Gibbs's reflective cycle?**

   Description, feelings, evaluation, analysis, conclusions, action planning

3. **What might be a drawback to using Gibbs's cycle within reflective practice?**

   It stops at the end of the reflective processes and does not proceed to the 'taking action' stage of the ERA cycle.

4. **What are the main differences between Gibbs's and Johns's frameworks?**

   | Gibbs | Johns |
   | --- | --- |
   | The framework arose from education | The model arose from clinical practice |
   | It focuses on the experience itself | It focuses on uncovering the knowledge behind the experience |
   | It is a reflective cycle consisting of six stages | It has a core question and a series of cue questions |
   | It focuses on learning from the incident | It focuses on the practitioner's intentions and actions |
   | It focuses on the individual's actions | It incorporates the actions of others present |

5. **What are Carper's types of knowing?**

   Empirics, ethics, personal, aesthetics

6. **What are Borton's three cue questions?**

   What? So what? Now what?

## Chapter 4

1. **What is the primary difference between the college environment and the practice environment?**

   The college's purpose is education; whereas the primary purpose in practice is to deliver a health-care service to the public.

2. **To whom do you have responsibilities in the clinical environment?**

   To yourself; to patients and their carers; to other staff and colleagues.

3. **What are your roles as a student in the practice environment?**

   To learn to be a safe and competent professional practitioner; to deliver care; to work as a team member.

4. **What is meant by 'self-empowerment'?**

   Taking responsibility for your own actions and enabling yourself to achieve for the future.

5. **What are the different types of learning opportunities available in clinical practice?**

   Learning from others; learning from different clinical placements; learning from events; learning through achievement of course competencies and learning outcomes; learning from your own interests and needs.

6. **What is meant by the term 'socialisation processes'?**

   How we learn to fit into different social situations and function within our profession. They include the language we use, the ways in which we work, our attitudes, skills and professional attributes.

7. **How can we get the most out of the opportunities available for learning in practice?**

   By taking the time to reflect, analyse and plan.

# Chapter 5

**1. What is the difference between reflection-in-action and reflection-on-action?**

Reflection-in-action occurs while we are doing things and is largely unconscious. Reflection-on-action occurs after the event and is a deliberate activity.

**2. What is reflective writing?**

Reflective writing is writing for the purpose of learning from your experiences and identifying future action.

**3. What are the features of reflective writing?**

We write reflectively to:

● Achieve a purpose
● Order our thoughts
● Create a permanent record
● Be creative
● Develop our analytical skills
● Develop our critical thinking
● Develop new understandings and knowledge
● Show that we understand something.

**4. What are the two categories of reflective writing?**

Analytical and creative.

**5. How can you plan to write safely?**

Safe writing involves:

● Setting your own rules
● Establishing the purpose of your reflection
● Selecting your own models and frameworks
● Retaining control over who sees your writing and what they see
● Storing it in a safe place
● Planning to complete the reflective cycle.

# Chapter 6

**1. What are the benefits of reflecting with others?**

They can take a more objective stance to something that has happened to you:

● They may ask questions that you have not thought of yourself
● They may offer a different way of seeing things
● They can act as a sounding board for your ideas
● They can validate your thoughts about a situation
● They may help you to put events into a different context
● They bring their own knowledge and experiences to the situation which may help your understanding
● They may offer alternative courses of action to those you have come up with.

**2. What different groups of people could you choose to reflect with?**

Family, friends and colleagues; staff in the clinical environment; educational staff.

**3. What issues do you need to think about before starting to reflect with others?**

To establish the purpose of the encounter; to consider the nature of the relationship; to set boundaries and ground rules; to consider the risks of reflecting with others; to consider the professional and ethical implications.

**4. How can you make the most of reflecting with others?**

● We can use the different relationships that we have with others for different kinds of reflection, remembering that one-to-one reflection has a different nature from group reflection.
● Forward planning before any reflective encounter with others will ensure that our own needs are met.
● Remember that the primary responsibility for the student's learning within reflective encounters lies with the student.

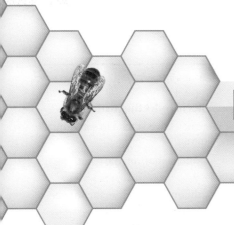

# Index